To MAUREE

GW00871206

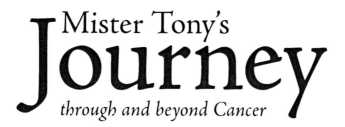

Mister Tony's Journey
through and beyond Cancer

Tony Power

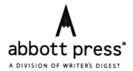

abbott press®
A DIVISION OF WRITER'S DIGEST

Mister Tony's Journey through and beyond Cancer

Copyright © 2012 Tony Power

All rights reserved. No part of this book may be used or reproduced by any means, graphic, electronic, or mechanical, including photocopying, recording, taping or by any information storage retrieval system without the written permission of the publisher except in the case of brief quotations embodied in critical articles and reviews.

Abbott Press books may be ordered through booksellers or by contacting:

Abbott Press
1663 Liberty Drive
Bloomington, IN 47403
www.abbottpress.com
Phone: 1-866-697-5310

Because of the dynamic nature of the Internet, any web addresses or links contained in this book may have changed since publication and may no longer be valid. The views expressed in this work are solely those of the author and do not necessarily reflect the views of the publisher, and the publisher hereby disclaims any responsibility for them.

Any people depicted in stock imagery provided by Thinkstock are models, and such images are being used for illustrative purposes only.

Certain stock imagery © Thinkstock.

ISBN: 978-1-4582-0281-9 (sc)
ISBN: 978-1-4582-0282-6 (e)

Library of Congress Control Number: 2012905022

Printed in the United States of America

Abbott Press rev. date: 7/9/2012

Table of Contents

Introduction

We must try to have a more holistic approach to our lives in general. We must try to eat the foods that heal our bodies.

Every body in some way is touched by cancer.

Some will die some will live. I chose to live and enjoy my life one day at a time.

Originally back in October 04 I was diagnosed with bilateral kidney cancer. I was given thirty days to live.

The shock alone nearly killed me. I lost one kidney and a piece of the other one. One year later I lost a piece of my right lung, and I thought I would never get well again but I did. In mid 09 I had brain surgery and I truly thought this was it, lights out for me. I was wrong again.

Every day that I live is a big bonus, and a blessing to me.

Over the years I have learned to calm my racing thoughts, my life is now very meaningful.

I thank the God of my understanding for every breath that I take, and for every day that I live.

I am happy to be who I have become. Cancer doesn't bother me it's only a word. It scared me at first but as time passed by; I embraced it and took ownership of it.

I have some bad days but I wait for the good ones and thank God they do come.

Chapter One:
The Journey Begins

I would like to start this by explaining; why I chose the word can-sir, instead of the proper spelling, it's because the word cancer doesn't scare me any more. I broke the word down, and to me it means I can sir-vive, you can- sir vive, and we can- sir vive.

It sounds like a big bully of a word but its not.

Where do I start and what do I say.....

It was October 2004 Boulder City, just a half hour from Las Vegas. I was supposed to celebrate my big 40th, and at the same time my friend Paul Fisher, was to celebrate his 92nd. I was so looking forward to it all, and in an instant life changed for ever. P. C. as I called him had arranged the whole trip.

He arranged for us, meaning his step daughter my partner (at the time) lets call her Mary, and her three kids to stay in his space house, commissioned by NASA for a prototype living accommodation unit that could be used on the moon.

Every thing in the house was ultra modern and high Tec; it was like some thing out of Star Trek;

The toilets cleaned themselves and the flooring hoovered itself. I may add "Wow" something else coming from where I came from.

It was a super experience. The first night there and Mary got very drunk, and wanted to go in the Jacuzzi; I didn't, this started a small few words, all of a sudden I was kicked in the left side just above the hip, it hurt a lot. I took a pain killer which did nothing to ease the pain. It was 3 in the morning Mary was asleep, she woke and all hell broke loose; the cops appeared and asked what all the noise was at three in the morning?

They asked was anybody assaulted. I told them no, I fell getting into the Jacuzzi.

One of them said, "We will give you lift to the hospital just get yourself checked out."

I being Irish kind of internally grinned at this, but I went anyway and thank God and his blessed mother I did.

For a town of about 7000 people; wow what a hospital state of the art towards back in Ireland, thank God and his blessed mother again. As I lay there at 4 in the morning being prepped and having test after test I wondered what the …. My thoughts got deeper with every test; I was starting to get scared. Here I was on my own, or at least I thought so on the other side of the world in hospital. At 6am the top doctor on duty told me that there was something wrong with my kidney functions, and that there were golf ball size objects on my kidneys.

Oh shit is this can- sir.

He said, "I don't know but you'll have to see the specialist in Las Vegas first thing in the morning."

By 7am I did not want to ring Mary, so all as I could do was ring Theresa at the Fisher Space Pen company who was PCs personal secretary, and also an earthly angel, who guided me through rough storms in the past. She woke P.C. and he arrived at the hospital. From where I was lying I could see the hall way, and PC was hobbling down to me. It was a sight I will never forget till the day I die, the old man coming to help the young man. He asked me what was wrong. I told him what the doctor said, he said, "Don't worry Tony we'll sort it out some how now let's go for breakfast, and Theresa can sort doctors and specialist appointments for you."

Mary was woken and told of the situation, and within a short while she appeared on the scene. We all had breakfast and tried to make plans but we just had to wait to see the specialist.

We drove to Vegas where the specialist read the test results and preformed a few of his own, one which was horrible, he put gloves on and I think it's possible to guess the rest yourself.

The results were in and his exact words were, "**Mister Power you have can- sir on your two kidneys, and I feel if you don't get one out in less than 30 days you will die, and some serious work will have to be preformed on the other one, and you might not survive because the surgeries have to be preformed very close together.**"

Shit! I was devastated, pain, sorrow, loss, anger, fear all raised their ugly head. I said I was going for a smoke as I needed to be on my own to gather my thoughts. I walked out side and I sat on the foot path.

My cell phone suddenly rang and it was Mary's mother Maria, who I believe was another earthly angel. Theresa had phoned her and told her of my situation, Maria said, "Close your eyes right now and pour the blood of Jesus Christ over your kidneys Tony."

I did and I still do so today. That moment life changed for me in a deep simple spiritual way. I felt a deep internal rush through my whole body from my hair to my toes, and I know it wasn't an earthly feeling. I looked up at the cloudless Nevada sky, and I knew at that moment that if I wanted to survive I would have to establish self control and self direction in my life.

We left the oncologist and headed for lunch, I needn't tell you I could not eat at all. All I wanted was answers, why, what, where, and when did this begin, and how am I going to fix this horrible disease.

Chapter Two:
The Offer and the Help

Paul was a wise old man and he took me aside and said, "What ever it takes Tony I will sell the Fisher Space pen Company and we will buy you kidneys", and he sincerely meant it.

It still blows my mind away when I think of what he offered and how sincere he was. There was one condition and that was to tell nobody so I did not until now. I decided to decline his offer because at the time all that was on my mind was getting home to mother Ireland.

I also felt that it was more blessed to give rather then receive.

My earthly angel Theresa over the next few days arranged flights, and got in touch with my G.P. Doctor Mark Rowe in Waterford Ireland. Mark is the best at what he does. He is a wonderful human being, he has looked after me for the last twelve years, and I hope he will look after me for the rest of my life. Theresa arranged meetings with the surgeons in Ireland for the day that I would arrive home. What an angel thank God and his blessed mother.

So for me it was all panic and pain, with doom and gloom death and a coffin. My mind was shattered.

Mary had a lot of experience with can- sir; her mum had it a few times and survived it.

Lots of people in the Fisher Space pen factory knew lots of Indian medicine so they gave me lots of potions, and herbs and for some strange reason my mind was open to all offers.

My real journey in, life, discovery, and spirit, and in faith had just begun.

One of the first things I remember my mother saying as a child was. "Close your eyes and open your mouth and see what god sends you." As I closed my eyes she would slip a sweet of some kind in my mouth. As an adult what came to me was, close your mouth and open your eyes and ears see what God sends you.

I needed time to pray, something I always did on my own but didn't know why up till then. Oh boy did I pray from my, heart, soul, body and mind.

Mary bought me a lot of books, most on can- sir and some on healing from within, and a couple on meditation. Somehow I had to absorb all in these books, and nit pick away and look for the answers if there was any.

I was coming to a point where my brain was like a sponge, it was full and no more would or could fit in there. This happened real fast. I needed to chill and control my thoughts, and centre myself in the eye of the on coming storm.

The journey home to Ireland was coming fast and I was not at all ready for it. After all I was going straight to the hospital for surgery, and that day was the tenth of October 2004, (my 40th birthday) it seems such a long time ago now.

Theresa sprang into action and hired a people carrier for Mary and her kids and me to drive to Los Angelus, to get the flights home to Ireland. We had a few days in Vegas before we left.

P.C called me and asked me to come to his office, and one hour later I arrived there. He said, "Come for a walk with me Tony." We went to the car park and he gave me an envelope. He told me to tell nobody. As he left the car park, I opened the envelope there was 4,000 dollars in it. Straight away I went to him and said, what's this for? He said, "It's for you to enjoy and treat yourself before you go home, but don't tell any one."

Over the next few days I had a full body treatment, this was the first time in my life for me, and I enjoyed a massage, facial and a manacure. I was feeling uplifted but that was on the outside. The inside was a different kettle of fish. It felt like I was in a deep hole with no ladder to climb out. The abyss, the bottom, the end.

Where was I going to find the light, the hope, and the faith to carry on? I was totally out of touch with my soul and this was truly killing me off as time ticked by. Maria phoned me and told me to go shopping for new clothes. Don't spare the dollars she said, "Buy lots of p.js for hospital, and make sure you buy new clothes for when you're coming out of hospital Tony."

This was a pure moment of light for me it was like she was conditioning me to believe all would be well for me. Her small few words were words of grace, and courage, and wisdom. Now I realise why god gave us all two ears and two eyes and only one mouth, if he wanted us to talk all the time we would have two mouths.

Now I had to empty my mind from all negative thoughts, and fill it with positive thoughts and visions, if I wanted to survive this nasty little bug.

But it's not an easy thing being human for weakness shows its ugly head especially in the grip of can- sir.

Guilt, Blame, Helpless, Despair, Worthless, Mood swings, Anxiety, Nervousness, Worry, Suicidal thoughts, these are the basic ones and the dangerous ones. From my experience they must be overcome sometimes on a daily basis, and if daily doesn't work hourly, if hourly fails take it minute by minute.

I wondered what went wrong in my life was it my job my life style or my thought patterns. If I truly wanted to get well I would have to do a complete inventory of my life from my earliest memory till now. Not an easy thing when you're told you are dying.

I had to uncondition the conditioned.

I had to play my role in this drama of my life, but most of all I had to be honest with all my internal and external affairs, because I believed the truth would set me free and it did and still does.

I was looking for the enemy I wanted to fight back, and I was asking the God of my understanding for help. I asked for the patience to be patient and I think I was not let down. I felt I asked from deep within my heart and soul.

This new found patience led to a place of positive planning, and positive thinking. At this time I was compelled to read the holy bible. I had a copy and it was 150 years old, actually it was a mission bible I got at a flea market in Ireland years ago. First I just picked my way through it.

Parables and phrases were all that I could take in.

I was reading and tears flowed like water from the sink tap, this was a pure and positive thing as this was the first time I cried since the diagnosis. The tears were my first weapon against can- sir as a matter of fact probably my strongest.

Deep inside I was dreading going home to Ireland as I knew, our hospitals were not up to scratch with a lot of the worlds. But I learned since that the people who work in them are probably the best in the world at what they do; from the cleaners to the surgeons. I wanted to run away from the cellar of my mind or to vanish from existence, but there is no escape because it lives within and eats away at the body mind and soul.

It was the 7 of October 04. We all packed our bags and we were on the road by 11am. I had a nine hour drive ahead; it did not bother me because I was heading home to my mother land. The long drive kept my mind off the ugly future. About four hours into the journey the people carrier was heating up, eventually the stop light came on. I thought shit why now why me, after all it was a new people carrier with only 10,00km on the clock. I knew I had to stop and in the middle of the Mohave Desert, it wasn't the right place for man or animal. As I drove on I lifted my vision to the horizon and lo and behold, in the distance I could see a MacDonald's M sign sticking up out of the desert. This amazed me and I saw this as a temporary safe haven, and a chance to unwind. I phoned Theresa and told her we had broken down, she phoned the hire company and they said it would be 3 to 4 hours before they get there with a replacement car. We all went into MacDonald's and filled up on rubbish. I finished my big Mac meal and went outside for a smoke. I was sitting on the pavement for five minutes and this beautiful Harley Davison pulled up, the guy driving it was a big bearded man. I said, "Howareya" as we do in Ireland. The first thing he said to me was, "Your Irish." I replied yes. He said, "What are you doing in the middle of nowhere?"

He could see I was confused and bewildered, and tired by the look on my face. I sat on the pavement and told him my story he didn't seem shocked, he put his hand in his pocket and slipped out a card and gave it to me; it was the King of Hearts. As I looked at it shivers ran up the back of my neck and at that moment I knew I was not alone in my struggle.

He said, "When the time is right pass it on, do you understand." Yes I do I answered. He said to me, "You will be all right and stop worrying."
Somehow I believed him.
As he mounted his bike he winked at me. When he turned his back to drive off I could see his colours, he was a black sheep biker for Christ.

Was this a dream?
No it wasn't.

This was the beginning or the refuelling of my faith, and nobody can tell me any different. Three hours later the recovery truck arrived with a new people carrier. We transferred our bags and we were on the road again heading for Los Angelus again.

After about two hours of hard driving my sight picked up mountains far off in the distance I could make out the outline. These were the San Andres Mountains. It took about an hour to get to them and another hour to drive to the top. When I looked down the other side I was in shock. The sight was amazing but scary.
I could see the 101 sign for the great American highway running parallel with the bottom of the mountains.

There were six lanes on each side, and I was heading right down there to connect with it.
I put my can- sir to one side for the moment for I needed one hundred and ten percent of concentration to get to Los Angelus. It was also getting dark this made the drive harder.
I was not used to these big roads. They were a living nightmare. The roads back in Ireland were microscopic compared to this.

One hour later I made it to the city of Angel's. P.C and Theresa had arranged for us to stay in the poshest hotel, as a treat before the long journey home to Ireland.

Mary was from Los Angelus and had lots of friends there she said to me, "I will get a baby sitter for the kids and we will go for a meal."

My heart or mind wasn't in it but I went anyway. The meal was fantastic pork and black bean sauce Shit; it was like the last supper for me. We decided to go for a drink, and of all the places on earth we went to the House of Blues how ironic. I don't drink never really did, but I felt I needed a pint of the black stuff. When I got it; I lobbed it down in two gulps. This was a short break from my reality and my unsettled mind.

We got talking to some really nice people and decided to go for a cigarette. I told my story to one guy and he said, "Did you ever smoke pot." I said yes years ago.

He said, "Pot and can-sir go hand in hand and you should try it again." "It will relax your muscles and help switch off the thought process or at least slow it down."

He pulled a joint out of his shirt pocket and handed it to me. I lit it and started smoking it. After two pulls my head was spinning, my mouth was as dry as Death Valley, but I felt ok and totally relaxed.

Fear of the future had no place to live for my head was full of emptiness.

Void of all thought, it felt peaceful. I liked the feeling it produced. Mary and I left the House of Blues on Sunset Strip and walked back to the hotel.

By now the effects of the pot were wearing off and I was feeling sick in my belly. When I reached the hotel room I bolted to the loo and vomited my guts up. This felt good. It felt like I was vomiting my fear of the future away.

I went to bed that night and prayed from my heart and soul. I asked the god of my understanding to give me strength for my journey through and beyond can- sir. I slept like a baby that night. When I woke I felt refreshed and recharged. I was ready for the long journey home.

I was truly ready to carry my cross of life.

I believe accepting this cross would infuse me with strength of mind and confidence.

I believe if I carry it willingly some day it would carry me. It seemed like I was putting things together in my mind, but being human I wondered when I would fall apart. This was negative thought at its best.

I felt I had a million questions in my mind, and the only one that could answer them was me.

Time seemed to be distorted for me. I remember counting the hours left to catch the flight home; every minute seemed like an hour. As time ticked by I thought of my daughter Elaine and son Shane back home in Ireland, and how in the name of God was I going to break the news to them.

Mary said, "Pick up the phone now and talk to them, and break it softly and no drama or tears Tony."

I was so scared for their feelings I could not dial the numbers so Mary dialled for me. Shane answered and I told him what the oncologist said, he was fourteen at the time and he handled it very well for a kid his age.

Shane didn't seem to be worried, I think he knew his dad very well and he knew, I was a fighter and come hell or high water I would survive.

Elaine was different she shut down I could barely get a word out of her.

We had to be in the airport by twelve o clock, the flight was leaving at two p.m. I packed the bags and off we went. The trip home consisted of two flights the first one was to Atlantic City, and the second one was to Dublin Ireland. I slept like a baby all the way home, only waking to transfer flights. I woke an hour before landing and I felt refreshed and recharged. These feelings disappeared as the thoughts in my head roamed back to can- sir and Fear raised its ugly head again, and for want of a better word I was shitting my self.

Faced with life threatening surgeries it left my mind in a very insecure and unstable place. I wondered was my life going to be ever normal again, would I die? Would I live? And if I lived would I be cared for by others for what was left of my life. I think the fear was worse than the reality.

As the plane landed in Dublin I wondered had I brought this can- sir on my self, and if so could I shake it off my self.

I had no personal control over this situation but I knew I would have to hand it over to God, and soon if I wanted help from the world beyond ours.

I began to believe that my God can do for me what I can't do for my self. I realise now that faith, and hope, are impossible to achieve unless I hand it over to the God of my understanding.

Chapter Three:
The Big Show Down

Mary her kids and I got a taxi straight to the Mater Hospital.

Theresa suddenly phoned and said, "Tony be calm and patient and this will pass."

It's easier said than done when one is in the eye of the storm. All I wanted at this time was to speak to the surgeon.

The waiting was doing my head in. We sat out side the consulting room drinking coffee; we were there for about an hour. I was feeling very anxious, and this feeling was exhausting my mind. Suddenly the door opened and the surgeon's secretary called my name, this was it the big show down.

As we entered the room the surgeon introduced himself and his small team of two. His name was Mister Akiatar and he was of Indian origin. One of the other people in the room introduced himself as Mister Murphy from Waterford the same city that I was from; this made me feel good for some strange reason.

Mister Akiatar explained what was going to happen; all the pros and the cons were explained to me and surgery was scheduled for the next day. He said, "You're coming in now and we are starting you fasting straight away."

"No way!" came straight out of my mouth without even thinking. I said it's my big 40 today, and I need a week to celebrate because this could be my last birthday.

I told him I was going to get pissed and stoned for the week. I think he was more shocked than me. I told him I had to see my family in Waterford and spend some precious time with them. Mister Akiatar agreed and told me to go home and enjoy the week. He said, "Be back here next Thursday morning and start fasting as soon as you wake up."

Mary her three kids and I left the hospital and got a taxi all the way to Mary's house in County Wexford. It took four hours to get there. We all were shattered from the long journey home; all we could do that night was sleep. I woke at six in the morning; as I lay in bed all hell broke loose in my mind. I was full of negative shit. I could not control my thoughts.

Mary and her three children were still asleep. The Sun was starting to rise.

I got out of bed got dressed and went straight for the coffee pot and the cigarettes. As I sat there sipping away at my coffee and smoking cigarettes, my mind was in overdrive, it even went as far as my funeral.

My mind was not in a peaceful place that morning.

If I wanted victory over this can- sir and this mental suffering it caused me, I knew I would have to change my way of thinking.

It was 8 a.m. and I got up and drove to the dog home and collected Lana our dog. She was over excited to see me. Ten minutes later we arrived back at the house. I picked up her lead and off we went down the country road.

Lana kept nudging me on both sides, just above the hips.

She never did this before and it didn't take long for me to realise, she knew that there was something wrong with me. This amazed and amused me. We walked on and I could see the sun coming up over the tall country hedges it was a magnificent sight.

There were sheep in a field and horses in another one. It was so peaceful no people, no cars, no town, just me and nature.

This was the first time since diagnosis that I had time on my own, time to gather my thoughts and feelings. It was time to arm my self mentally and spiritually for what lay ahead.

I learned that morning to leave the past behind, forget about the future, and try keep my self in the here and now.

I learned if I keep digging up the past all I will get is dirt.

The future was like a cheque I would have to wait to have it cashed.

I realised that beautiful morning in October 04 that silence is the greatest element in which great things can be transferred into reality.

This was the first time I felt hope in my heart and a bit of peace in my mind.

That morning I asked for help from all the saints and angels in heaven, and all the holy men and women on earth. I believe and still do believe help came that wonderful day.

Lana and I slowly wandered back to the house.

My head was in the clouds, it was a wonderful feeling but I knew I had to get my head back to earth in order to get the practical things done.

Lana and I arrived back at the house Mary had a full Irish breakfast ready, the children were happy to be at home. There was a happy energy hovering about the house, it felt good and wholesome.

I ate my breakfast it was delicious.

In the early summer of 04 I had built a grotto in the corner of Mary's garden. I finished my breakfast and went straight to it. I knelt down and prayed with the rosary beads from my heart and asked for help.

At that moment I knew I had to inject peace into my blood, muscles, nerves, soul, and heart.

From that moment on I never felt alone, even when I was on my own.

I saw sorrow as a gift to exercise my mind for the journey ahead.

Deep inside I started to feel I could beat this monster called can- sir.

Little by little small spiritual insights were popping up in my mind. I think this was Gods way of waking me up and preparing me for the journey ahead.

It was ten in the morning, it was time to leave Wexford and head for my home town Waterford, which was a fifty mile drive away.

The drive home was very pleasant; the sun was shining through the scattered clouds. My mind was empty void of all thought. This was a bit of respite for my weary brain.

I was very happy to cross the bridge in Waterford City.

I drove straight to my home, and as soon as I entered the house I picked up the mail as I opened each envelope I was amazed. Five out of the ten letters were Mass cards, and four were get well soon cards. I realised there and then the power of other people's prayers. I felt peace and harmony, this was my cave it was also my personal house of prayer. I lit some candles and I knelt down and asked the God of my understanding for strength to carry on this journey of mine. As tears flowed, some how fear and terror did not reside in me at that moment. I was willing to accept the path ahead, and even make my own path. My inner self was starting to accept the road ahead.

I lay down on the couch and prayed with the rosary beads, something I did for years, I must have drifted off to sleep. I was woken by the door bell I answered it. It was my son Shane. He seemed to be upset and he was waffling on.

I told him the bad days would pass and tomorrow was another day. I was so overjoyed to be with him it gave me a sense of belonging, a sense of being connected to humanity.

I thought if I die in surgery the gift I will leave behind is my son and daughter Elaine.

It was three in the afternoon; it was time to go to Doctor Rows practice. Shane and I got in the car. I said to Shane, do you want to come with me to the doctors.

He said, "No" some how I understand how he felt. As I dropped him at his mum's house, Elaine was sitting on the front door steps.

Elaine was born with cerebral palsy. I met her mum when Elaine was only one year old.

As Elaine got older she was showing no signs of walking.

The diagnosis at that time was that Elaine would never walk. I refused to believe this. Elaine's mum and I had heard from a good friend about a special clinic in Budapest in Hungary. The only thing was it was very expensive. We got permission from the police to fund raise. We raised thirty five thousand Irish pounds and got Elaine to the clinic in Hungary three times, she did very well there. When we got home to Ireland I took it upon my self to carry on with the exercises that we learned. Today Elaine walks on crutches and refuses to use a wheel chair. Here was somebody who gained strength and courage as time passed by.

I said God bless and take care to Shane and Elaine.

I drove to Doctor Rowe. I was only waiting for five minutes before he called me in to his office. I was pleased to see him. Mark, (Dr Rowe) asked me, was I all right.

I replied, no I don't think so my head won't slow down.
He said, "You are in need of some spiritual and emotional healing."
I said it feels like I am in the middle of a night mare and I haven't woke up yet. It feels like a death sentence. I told him I was in a disturbed state of mind, and I told him how scared, shocked, and confused I was deep inside.

Mark said, "You will cross many bridges on your journey but don't cross them until you're ready to cross them."

With the best intentions Mark offered me some diazepam. I said no, I will face this without diazepam. "Well he said you've crossed the first bridge."

I had taken diazepam and strong pain killers years ago after a bad motor bike crash. I hit a horse head on; my head was so messed up from tablets. I lost my marriage, there was no talking to me at that time in my life, and I would not listen to any body. My behaviour towards others was disgusting and disturbing.
I knew deep inside tablets and being blotto was not going to help me with this can- sir saga.

Mark gave me his cell phone number and said, "The line is open for you twenty four seven."
I felt a sense of comfort as I left his office that day.
I went straight home to my cave. I phoned Mary in Wexford and told her how tired I was and that I was going to bed. She said, "Did you talk to your parents yet?"
I said no, and I am not going to until tomorrow.

Here I was all on my own; it was six in the evening.
I turned the television on it was a waste of time. I could not concentrate or focus on it, for my thoughts were regularly drifting back to can- sir.

I put some instrumental music on and turned the stereo up full blast, the house was rocking. I danced around the house that evening, and I really enjoyed being on my own. For brief moments while I was dancing can- sir was not present in my mind.

I turned the music off and lay down on the couch; I drifted off into a deep sleep.

I was suddenly woken by the door bell, I answered it, my son Shane was there, and he said, "I am staying with you tonight dad."

I was pleased to have somebody with me, we spent hours talking and laughing.

I went to bed at eleven thirty. I knelt down to say my prayers and I found it hard to stop praying. In my prayer I was not asking for help. I was thanking the God of my understanding for getting me this far through life. I grabbed my rosary beads and slipped into bed.

As I lay there I was recalling the past and how my mum dragged us all too mass on Sundays.

She also told us to say one million Hail Marys, and we would get a bigger present from Santa for Christmas. I don't know if she did this just so she could get a bit of peace and quiet. She had her hands full rearing seven of us, as dad spent some of the early years in the pub.

As I lay in my bed saying the rosary over and over my mind wandered. I was still praying but yet my mind was in different places, places of peace and harmony.

I guess this was some form of meditation. Eventually I drifted off to sleep. I woke at about seven and my mind was in a state of peace and rest.

I cooked a big wholesome Irish breakfast, loads of fat just the thing for Shane and person with can- sir.

I had a big bath and I decided to drive to Mount Mellary.

Chapter Four:
Mini Spiritual Retreat

Mount Mellary is the home of the Benedict monks in North West Waterford. It's about forty miles from Waterford city. I dropped Shane home and I headed for Mellary. It took me about an hour to drive there.

Just a mile or so before Mount Mellary there is a grotto of Our Lady. When I was a small boy there were moving statues all over Ireland, this was a hot spot, and people flocked there from all parts of the country.

My mother arranged a bus journey to the grotto.

We all had a wonderful time, every person there was praying.

As a young child I felt a sense of peace there.

As a grown man with can- sir I wanted that sense of peace in my life again.

I arrived at the grotto at 11 in the morning. I parked the car in the car park and crossed the road to the grotto.

To my amazement there was not a single person there.

I knelt down and asked the powers that be for some help.

I can remember very clearly asking for the strength of mind and the courage of heart to fight this disease that was destroying me.

I left the grotto and drove the mile or so to the monks Abbey. I parked the car and walked around the beautiful gardens.

There was a sense of peace there. My soul was seeking a place of healing, silence, and tranquillity.

I left the gardens and went into the chapel in the Abbey. I sat down and prayed for a message or a sign that I was on the right road.

I did not have to wait long.

Out of the corner of my eye I could see a monk approaching me. He sat in the aisle opposite me and acknowledged my presence with a nod.

I felt compelled to talk to him.

As the monk was leaving the chapel I called him to the side, and told him briefly about my journey so far.

I asked him could he administer the last rights, he said "Yes come with me."

I followed him though a maze of corridors, as I walked behind him I could sense this was a place of spirituality and wisdom.

Eventually we arrived at his small humble office.

We entered and sat down.

I told him my whole life story from my earliest memory up till now. He did not speak once he just sat there listening to me.

When I was finished speaking he took a big black book out of a book case and placed it on the table.

He opened the book and to my amazement the page was page 117.

I was given a book in America it was a book about Essiac, which was the Native American cure for can- sir, the last page in this book was 117.

I told the monk of this coincidence he said, "Have you got the book with you."

Yes I said it's in the boot of the car, I didn't get the time to unpack every thing yet.

He said, "Can you go and get it."

I left and got the book and returned to his office.

I showed him a paragraph that I had underlined.

It was proof that three of the four herbs used to make up Essiac were used at the Last Supper.

He said to me, "O my God, the Holy Spirit is guiding you and it's up to you whether you accept this guidance or not."

The monk then gave me the last rights and anointed me with the holy oil.

As I was leaving the last thing he said to me was, "When we listen, God speaks and when we obey, God works wonders."

My head was in the clouds I felt good.

I drove back to the grotto there was still nobody there I had the whole place to myself.

I sat and prayed for half an hour. When I was leaving I filled some bottles with holy water to bring home with me. I also splashed my body with the water.

I got into my car and it would not start, after about ten minutes she fired up, but the fuel gauge was indicating empty. This was bothering me big time because I had put thirty euro in the tank before I left, and the nearest petrol station was about ten miles away.

As I drove off I switched the radio on and I could not believe what was playing, it was George Michael and the song was YOU GOT TO HAVE FAITH.

This freaked the head out of me.

I had to stop the car and try to calm myself.

I was so glad I was on my own that day, because I burst into buckets of tears. They were not tears of pain they were tears of pure joy and bliss. I noticed that the fuel gauge returned to where it should have being. I wondered in the name of God, what was going on. I wondered does God mess around with electronics.

To me these were signs that I was on the right path, my path.

I drove on.

After about ten minutes I started to feel itchy all over my body, and small blisters appeared everywhere.

Now I was really starting to get scared. I was imagining all sorts of negative things.

I drove on and decided to take the coast road to Waterford.

The views of the ocean and the mountains were fantastic, they seemed to energise me. Somehow the rash all over my body didn't bother me at that time.

I felt at peace until I came to Waterford.

I went straight to the Waterford Regional Hospital and proceeded to the oncology out patients department.

I was as red as a Wexford strawberry, even down to my private parts.

The nurse there called me in to her room and did my blood pressure. As she did this I actually could feel every vain in my body expanding and swelling up. She said, "Mister Power your blood pressure is normal." This amazed and confused me; it sure didn't feel like every thing was normal. I felt like I was burning from the inside out.

The nurse said, "Stay here we are going to get the dermatologist to have a look at you."

As I sat waiting fear crept in, I wondered was this it? Were my kidneys failing, and would I even make it to surgery.

After about twenty minutes the door opened and the dermatologist walked in. He spent five minutes examining me, and than he told me it was scabies.

I was not going to sit there arguing with his silly stupid misdiagnosis.

I lost faith in him instantly.

I wouldn't trust him to put a plaster on a scratch.

He left the room and the nurse came in and gave me a tube of cream and said, "Put it on three times a day."

I said thank you and I left the room.

On the way out of the hospital I dumped the tube of cream in the bin.

As it was getting on in the day I headed straight home.

When I got there I just crashed out on the couch and drifted off into a deep sleep.

It seemed that every time I went to sleep I didn't have to worry about can-sir.

I woke at about nine o clock that evening.

The rash and blisters had all disappeared except for a few blisters on my hands and feet.

I could not fathom what went on that day.

It was beyond the thoughts of my rational mind.

I phoned Mary and told her the events of the day, she seemed not surprised she said, "Just accept the events of the day as something special."

I lit some candles and turned off the lights as my thoughts deepened I began to cry, tears flowed like never before, it was like a dam busting. I began to think, everybody's life is made up of sorrowful and joyful events that are beyond our control. I wondered what was broken in me, and how did it get broken? How could I fix it?

I realised that evening that the wounded child in me was missing something, missing love. I always had lots of love to give to others but none to give to my self.

I began to be conscious of the wounded child within me. The child in me had lots of painful memories, they were sorrowful and emotional.

I knew that evening that the child in me would have to be nourished in order to give me a fighting chance against this deadly disease called can- sir.

I felt as if all my life I had hidden a part of myself from society and from myself.

I blew the candles out and phoned Shane and Elaine. I wished them good night and God bless. I told them how much I loved them.

I also phoned Mary and told her the same thing. It was eleven o clock; it was time to go to bed.

I went to my bedroom and knelt down beside the bed and said my prayers.

After ten minutes or so I got into the bed and continued praying, this time I wasn't praying for me. I was praying for all the people in my life. I asked the God of my understanding to ease the emotional upset of the people that are close to me. As I prayed I could feel the stresses of the day evaporating from my mind, it seemed I was becoming less worried about the events ahead.

I drifted into a deep sleep. For me this deep sleep was a place void of all thoughts. I feel it was a place where god was energising me for the journey ahead.

I woke at seven thirty. I felt like somebody had spiked me with tranquilisers. I jumped into a cold water shower, and this reversed the tranquillised feelings I was having.

It was Wednesday morning; the first surgery was scheduled for Friday afternoon.

I poured three cups of coffee into me and sure enough I was ready for the day.

It was time to tell my parents.

My mum and dad had split up twenty five years ago, so I had to go to them separately and tell them the news.

First I went to mums house, as I entered I could see she was very upset, she got up out of the chair and hugged me very tightly and said, "Mary phoned me late last night and told me what is going on."

Mum put the big Irish breakfast on and we sat down and talked about prayers and healing. She told me that all her friends were praying for me and that it's going to be all right, some how I believed her even though she was upset.

My mum cuddled me in her arms, and tears flowed from both of us, like a river in full flood. It felt like I was a baby again in the arms of the woman who brought me into this world.

She told me to be calm and keep praying no matter what happens.

She told me that she was going to have mass said for me, and that God never left her down.

I cuddled into her arms again, and told her I was heading off to see my dad.

My mum wished me well, and said, "I will see you in the hospital in Dublin after your surgery." I said Please God and his blessed Mother, you will.

I left my mums house, and drove to my dad's house.

As I walked up the steps I was apprehensive and nervous.

I rang the bell and there was no answer. I went to the side gate and called out dad, he called back, "Who's that?" I said it's Tony.

He opened the side gate and we went into the back kitchen. He knew by the look on my face that there was something wrong.

He said, "Tony what's up?" I said Dad let's sit down; I have some bad news to tell you.

I told him while I was in America I was diagnosed with bilateral kidney can-sir, and that they gave me about thirty days to live.

Well he nearly fell off his chair.

He said, "Parents are supposed to die before their children."

I replied Dad I am still here, and I am going to give it my best effort to get well again!

As I said this, deep within my heart I realised that there is more to this than the physical world.

I left my dads house that day, and I left him in a state of shock and confusion.

Chapter Five:
The Mystery in the Mountains

I drove to Shane's mum's house and asked Shane to come with me to the Mahon Falls, which is up in the Commragh Mountains in west Waterford.

He said, "No dad, call me on the way back."

I left Shane

And I drove straight to the mountains. I drove as high as I could drive and stopped the car. I got out of the car and put my Wellie boots on and started to climb to the top. Half way up I was starting to puff and pant I was out of breath, and so I stopped and sat down.

I had my Rosary beads with me, and I felt this was the right time to pray and connect with the child that was lost and hurt a very long time ago.

I was about four thousand feet above sea level. I was sitting on a wide and deep ledge.

It was early October the temperature was near zero degrees. It was very cold and frosty.

The clouds were drifting past my face.

The wind was howling past my ears.

In the gaps in the clouds, I could see the land below. In the far off distance, I could see the ocean.

As I sat there my head trawled through a whole volume of emotions and feelings, from terrifying ones to uplifting ones.

I gradually became less worried about can- sir; I could feel the stresses of life gradually evaporating from my mind.

This was a critical moment for me.

I was in a place where I could shout out at the top of my voice and nobody could hear me, and that's exactly what I did.

I screamed at the top of my voice at God. I screamed at my parents. I screamed at my brothers and sisters. I screamed at my friends, and most important I screamed at me.

I had saved up all my hurt and anger over a period of my life, and these were all the principal hang-ups in my life.

I realised I had a shit load of emotional baggage that caused me and others a lot of pain over the years, and if I didn't dump it, it would keep dumping back on me.

I made a conscious decision that day to let the hurt of the past vanish into the universe.

I thought my history was my destiny, but now I know better.

That day on the mountains was the start of me disarming all my internal battles.

Here I was sitting on a mounting humbling myself to the truths and lies of my life.

I was adamant that fear or sorrow would not have the last word.

I decided to pray the rosary before my climb back down the mountain.

I gripped my beads tightly in my right hand.I prayed deeply from my heart and soul.

Really I was praying and looking for a spontaneous remission, in other words I was looking a miracle.

Suddenly out of nowhere the wind raised its velocity, and my hat blew of my head, and drifted down the mountain.

I watched the hat drifting down, and when it hit solid ground, and at that very moment the hairs on the back of my neck stood up, and a shiver ran down my spine.

I felt as if there was somebody with me, I was totally creped out but somehow I was not afraid.

It was getting on in the evening, and it was time to climb down the mountain.

On my way down the mountain, I wondered about all sorts of heavenly things. Things like Guardian Angels, healing Angels, messenger Angels and saints and holy men and women.

I felt totally safe wrapped up in these thoughts.

When I reached the bog below the mountain, I searched and found my hat.

I put it on my head and veered off towards my car.

I was about a hundred yards away from the car, when I noticed a bird on the bonnet of the car.

I slowly walked closer to the car. I did not want to scare the bird off.

At about twenty meters, the bird flew up in to the sky.

I intuitively knew it was a dove. My eyes followed him until he disappeared over the top of the mountain.

I was shaken by this event, for I knew that the dove

Is the universal symbol of the Holy Spirit.

Deep inside I knew this was a sacred event.

I knew I was on the right path.

As I walked over to the car I noticed something on the wind screen, and to my amazement it was a small yellow flower.

I picked it up and smelt it, it was a Devine smell.

I looked all around; there wasn't a car or a person in sight.

The place was empty and had being since I got there.

My human mind tried to figure this out but it was beyond my comprehension.

I got into the car, and the first thought that entered into my mind was.

Tony, don't be overwhelmed by fear and terror of the future, what begins in sorrow and pain ends in joy and Serenity.

As I drove off down the mountain, I felt like death had no hold on me.

It was six thirty in the evening.

I was driving towards Waterford it seemed, I was slowly getting in touch with my inner calmness.

It seemed that the can- sir had come to the surface in order to heal the wounded child in me.

An hour later I collected Shane from his mum's house and drove to Mac Donald's.

We sat in the car park and filed ourselves up with junk food.

I drove Shane home and said goodbye. I told him no matter what happens; I will love him till the end of time.

I hugged him close to my chest, as if it was for the last time I would ever hug him on earth.

Chapter Six:
The Journey to Wexford

I drove off and an immense amount of tears streamed down my face.

It was Wednesday evening time for surgery was ticking away.
I was feeling upset and tired.
I went straight home and sprawled out on the sofa, my breathing was irregular and my heart beat was all over the place.

Suddenly the phone rang, it was Mary and I was happy to hear her voice, it seemed to soothe my racing mind.
Mary said, "Have you packed your bits and pieces for hospital." I replied No I am going to do it as soon as I get off the phone.
Mary also told me that Theresa had phoned from America, and that she had booked a hotel for ten days, So Mary could have a bit of comfort while she was in Dublin tending to me.

I packed a small few things and put them in the car.
I locked the house up and drove off.
As I was driving, I looked back and wondered would I ever see my home or children again.

This thought scared the living day light out of me.
As I crossed the bridge in Waterford anxiety crept into my mind. After about ten minutes driving my mind eventually settled down.
It just felt good to be on my own.
It was just me and my higher power, having a good old one to one.

I asked God to look after the people that I love, and give them strength to cope with what ever was going to happen in the future to me.

I pulled into a filling station for some coffee and a smoke.

I realised there and then, I was offering myself to God and I was slowly surrendering to his will.

I asked God for the strength to stand fast and not give way under the stress of can-sir.

I wished for the opportunity and the ability to follow and accept his will.

I realised I had to have faith in my own path, and push true the storms of life.

By now I had a lot of faith in the power of my prayers.

Especially in the prayers to Our Lady, the mother of God, the queen of the universe.

I finished my coffee, and proceeded on my journey to Mary's house in County Wexford.

I picked my Rosary Beads up from the passenger seat and I prayed continually until I got to Mary's house.

I parked the car by the front gates and got out.

Lana jumped the gate and landed next to my feet. I could tell by her giddiness that she was well pleased to see me.

She licked my face and jumped all over me.

I told her to calm down but she would not listen to me.

Lana started nudging me on my left side just above my hip. It was obvious to me that Lana sensed; this was going to be the site of my first surgery.

Mary came to the gate and squashed me with a big hug.

We both went into the house and had some coffee.

Mary gave me some candles and flowers that she had bought in Wexford town, while I was in Waterford.

Mary said, "Tony you know what to do with them."

Instinctually I knew that they were for the grotto of our Lady in the garden.

I finished my coffee and walked up the garden to the grotto. I put the flowers at the feet of the statue of Our Lady. I lit the candles and sat down on the bench.

It was very dark that night; there was no moon in the sky.

The stars were like souls in Heaven.

My thoughts were deepening.

I thought if I want to see the light I must be in the dark.

I was truly in the dark.

I could see that my life was a mesh of sorrow and joy.

I realised,

I must look for the benefits of all my sorrows.

I was not going to let despair destroy and steal my courage and hope.

I was adamant to hold on to my faith come hell or high water.

That night I felt I was like a little orphan, under the shelter of God and his angels.

Words could not express how I was feeling deep in my Soul.

I told God that night if he wanted me, he could have me now. It felt like I was truly ready to go home.

So far my short inward journey forced me to look at both the light and dark side of myself and my life.

I think all of us live our lives with a bit of light and darkness, love and fear, and weakness, and strengths.

Personally Fear was the big one for me, fear that I would have to primarily rely on the grace of God for healing and well being.

If I was going to live after surgery I knew things would have to change. I could not allow myself to live on a superficial level any more.

I knew that night I would have to live on a spiritual level, for what was left of my life on this planet.

I felt that my soul some how was being harvested and nourished by God.

I had to satisfy the needs of my soul, and the only way to do this was to keep in contact with the God of my understanding.

My relationship with God was getting stronger by the hour.

It seemed like God was waiting patiently for me to discover my true self, and the Devine presence within me.

I was amazed by the amazing transformation of my thoughts.

My tired weak spirit was starting to be replenished and refreshed.

Even though my mind was still in an anxious and panicky mode, I felt I was at a place of deep comfort within my soul.

No matter what happened over the next couple of months, I felt like my soul was earning credits or points for entry through the pearly gates.

Just before I left the grotto I had a few moments of consultive reflections with God, and I realised that his guidance was infallible guidance.

Now it felt like I could trust my inner self to be led to a life of freedom and release.

This felt like a personal cleansing that would benefit my spiritual growth.

The mental paralyses I felt when I was diagnosed in America was evaporating into nothingness.

I understood that if my hope failed all hell would break loose.

I had to hold on tightly to the small bit of hope that was infused in me.

Suddenly Mary arrived at the grotto she sat with me and we prayed the Rosary together. We both got a sense of peace from this.

Mary said, "Tony its half past eleven and you're starting fasting at twelve, come down to the house and have something to eat."

I followed Mary to the house and she said, "What would you like to eat."

I wasn't very hungry so we just had carrot cake and Earl Grey tea.

When we finished Mary said, "I am off to bed."

I wasn't tired, so I told Mary that I was going to sit in the bird garden for a while.

Mary said, "It's cold out there, do yourself a favour and fire up the garden stove, and stop worrying about tomorrow."

I replied, easier said than done.

Mary went off to bed, and I went out the back door to the bird garden where the stove was.

I lit the stove with old news paper and sticks.

After about five minutes the fire was starting to take off, so I put some wooden blocks on it.

I sat down on the swinging bench. I tried to gather my thoughts. My mind was away with the fairies, I could not concentrate on any of my thoughts.

Suddenly I heard a lot of scratching sounds coming from the inside of the back door.

Obviously it was Lana wanting to go for pe pe.

I opened the back door and Lana shuffled her way out past me, she did her pe pe, and jumped up on the swinging bench.

I told her to get down, but she wasn't having any of it.

I physically tried to remove her, but she kept jumping back up on the bench.

Eventually I gave into her, and I sat down on the bench beside her.

Lana put her head on the left side of my lap and stayed dead still. I felt like she was comforting me in her own little way.

As I stared at the fire my thoughts were deepening.

I was trying to understand the emotional, mental, physical, and spiritual, effects that can- sir was revealing to me.

That night I saw can- sir as the enemy of my life.

I was forced to confront my mortality.

Ultimately I had to deal with this on my own.

I was not going to let my mind believe, that I was not able to cope with the stress that cans- sir was causing me.

I think can sir- can be a soul destroying experience, and it can take away from the purpose and meaning of life.

The stress of can- sir is like a vicious circle, it's like a trap that can force you into negative feelings, and it can diminishes ones ability to cope with every day duties and chores.

As I sat there I felt it was vital to tap into all the spiritual forces and resources, within me and outside me.

I felt like I had to draw on my deepest resources, and the deepest one in my armoury was God.

Mary's house was about three miles from the ocean, and in the stillness of the night I could hear the ocean crashing against the beach. I guess the tide was in and it would go out, as sure as night meets day.

These thoughts took the edge off the storm within me. The light house in the distance was beaming its light all over the land. It relaxed my mind to know that the light would return to me, all as I had to do was wait for it.

By now the fire was starting to go out, and Lana was snoring. I woke Lana up and we went straight into the house. Lana went straight to her wicker basket and she went back to sleep straight away.

I went to the sitting room and sat down on the couch in the dark.

I really needed to go to sleep, but my mind would not switch off. It was racing away with itself.

I asked the God of my understanding to show me the way to find joy, peace, and freedom.

I asked to be healthy whole and free from this can- sir.

I needed guidance support and power beyond my own.

I found strength in admitting my powerlessness to God.

Nevertheless I had to accept all that was happening to me, was Gods will for me for the salvation of my soul.

It was like God was believing in me until I could find the strength to believe in myself.

All my life I felt a sense of worthless, inadequacy, and inferiority, and low self-esteem.

I believe these feelings were infused in me, in my family life as a child.

I was seeking the willingness to make amends to myself before my surgeries.

I began to ask what can- sir is trying to tell me about my self and my past.

It was obvious to me that I would have to set things right before it was all too late.

It seemed like all the suffering I endured all my life was contained in me and it had manifested itself as can- sir.

It felt like I had two faces all my life, one for the world and one for myself in private.

I was slowly freeing myself from my cocoon of limited thinking.

I was gathering my power through insights and pure love.

These feelings and insights, over the last couple of weeks felt like I was starting an apprenticeship, an apprenticeship within my soul.

I looked at the clock it was three in the morning I was ever so tired. I put my feet up on the couch and started to pray the Rosary, and before long I drifted off into a deep sleep.

Lana stuck her snout into my face and woke me up at about seven o clock. My first thought was hospital, the second was surgery, and I wondered what hand will guide me through this ordeal.

Mary and her three children were still asleep, so I stayed very quiet around the house. It was still dark out and Lana was at the door, it was pe pe time for her. I picked her lead up and we both headed off into the darkness.

As we were walking the old country roads, the sun was starting to rise and show its beams. The negative part of me was wondering, was this the last time I would see the sun rising.

I knew there and then, that self defeating fear would not help me in my quest for freedom from this thing they call can- sir.

Lana and I sat on a grass verge beside the old Wexford and Waterford railway tracks.

The time and place was right for me to let go and shed tears, and I began to cry. This crying was different than before, it seemed like forty years of tears needed to be shed.

It felt like every single cell in my body was shedding tears. Lana licked every tear from my face that very special morning.

I was now starting to feel spiritually flexible, and trusting in my God and the queen of the universe.

I wondered would this story have a happy ending.

If it didn't, it would not matter because I made my peace with my self, and with my God.

I felt that my way of thinking had changed and because of this, I felt I could possibly out live my original prognosis.

By now the sun was moving higher in the blue sky, and Lana and I headed back to the house.

When we got there Mary and the kids were up and about.
Mary told me to pack the rest of my stuff for hospital.

Mary's mum had told me while I was in America to buy clothes for going into hospital, and more for when I was coming out. I spent eight hundred dollars out of the money that P.C. gave to me, on the best of clothes and p.jays and here I was packing as if I was going on a foreign holiday. A foreign holiday to combat Death.

Mary and I decided earlier on to get the eleven o clock train from Wexford town to the hospital in Dublin.
Mary had arranged for Florence, the grand mother of her children to mind them while we were away in Dublin.

Florence arrived at ten o clock, and Mary gave her a list of things to do for the next week or so.
Mary and Florence were chatting away.

I put the cases in the boot of the car, and I walked up to the Grotto.
I knelt down and said a short prayer for hope.
Suddenly my mind was fixated on the word hope.
I figured out in my brain, the word hope means hoping when everything seems hopeless. This was an opportunity to practise the grace of hope.

As I left the Grotto tears streamed down my face.
There was a certain feeling to these tears; it felt like they were tears of empowerment, or tears of hope.
I wiped my eyes with the sleeve of my jumper, just like a small child would wipe his nose with his sleeve.

Chapter Seven:
Train Journey

Now it was time for Mary and me to part.

Mary hugged her children and said, "Good bye."

I gave the children a group hug and told them I loved them, and I would see them next week.

Lana was sitting on the front porch, she looked ever so sad. I went over to her and lay down on the ground beside her.

She snuggled her snout into my left side, and licked me all over my face.

I got up of the ground and said good bye and God bless to Florence and the children.

Mary and me got in the car and drove off.

As we drove away I waved at the children, and silent tears flowed and engulfed my mind.

I was feeling sad but positive and emotional.

Mary was driving so I could sit back and try to enjoy the journey into Wexford train station.

Half way there Mary stopped at a filling station for petrol cigarettes and coffee.

Mary put the petrol in the car, and I went in to the shop to pay and get the coffee and cigarettes.

I was starving with the hunger so I bought some apple slices. I paid for everything and got back in the car.

Mary had a strange look on her face. She said, "Tony what in the name of God are you doing with cakes, have you forgotten your supposed to be fasting."

I said, O my God I did forget.

Mary took the apple slices and put them on the back seat of the car.

She said, "Out of sight out of mind."

We sat in the filling station and sipped our coffee and smoked a couple of cigarettes.

Mary reached over and took my hand into hers and said, "Don't be afraid, I have a strange feeling that you will be all right."

We drove off and within twenty minutes we were at the train station.

Mary parked the car in the long term car park.

I got out and took the bags from the boot of the car.

Mary locked the car and we walked to the ticket office.

Mary purchased two monthly return tickets for us.

I asked Mary did she want coffee, "Of course" she replied. I slipped across the road to O'Brien's sandwich bar and purchased two large coffees with an extra shot of coffee in each one.

I returned to the train station and sat down on a bench beside Mary, and gave her the coffee.

It was three minutes to eleven o clock, and I could hear the train coming down the track.

I stood up and looked to my right side and I could see the train plodding towards us.

This was it I knew there and than, that my real journey in life and discovery had begun.

The train pulled up at the platform.

We boarded the train and sat down.

I realised that no matter who was with me or not with me at the end of the day, I was going to have to face this on my own.

The reality was that this can- sir was mine, and mine alone. It was my cross and the only one that was capable of carrying it was me.

As the train pulled away from the station I was feeling full of anxiety and tension.

My mind would not settle, my heart beat was racing and I was sweating all over.

I was starting to get very impatient and insecure within myself.
I was faced with losing my life, and I could not run away from this.

This was my reality, and I wondered when I would give way under the weight of all this pressure.

I know now that in the uncertainty of life lays the drama of life.

I wondered how many more chances, happy chances I would get in life.

I was feeling frustrated trapped and under pressure. I figured out that if I wanted these feelings to vanish, I would have to attain great emotional and spiritual strength. I secretly wished somebody would wave a magic wand and make all this can-sir shit disappears.
But in the real world this was not going to happen.
I had to be realistic and leave my body in the hands of modern science.

I understood that the surgeons would do the work, and God and I would have to do the healing.

Nothing was predictable on this journey.
It's interesting how often in life I undervalued the importance of the spiritual realm.

Time seemed to be a major factor in my mind.
I secretly wondered how much I had left,
And how would I spend it wisely.

I had being so busy with others all my life, I rarely had time to be quiet and find a deep inner stillness.
Because I had no stillness in my mind I felt my soul was out of balance with the universe.

In order to be whole again, I needed to integrate the spiritual and emotional and psychological elements of my life.

As the train plodded on I wondered how I could dump this nightmare. I felt like I needed to detach from the events ahead of me.

I hoped that in time the confusion within me would be converted to clarity.

Deep inside I was feeling a mysterious co-operation between my soul and my heart.

I realised there and than that I had grown in some strange way.

I wondered would God rescue me, or would the doctors rescue me, or would I rescue me from this horrible thing called can- sir. Or would all three have a part to play in it.

By now I was starting to identifying the pending surgeries as a form of healing.

In a strange perverse way now I was looking forward to the surgeries.

Now my mind was starting to generate positive thoughts. It was like a shift in my attitude and outlook towards life in general.

I was starting to build control over my can- sir and it sure felt good and wholesome.

Really I was surrendering unconditionally to God, and it was up to me whether I made it easy on myself or hard on myself.

The lack of certainty was not going to scare me.

I was learning things from my experiences, and I wondered would it be possible to help others some day in the future.

I know now that the opportunity for spiritual growth is open to every single person on this planet that we all call home.

As the train plodded on towards Dublin, I started to take a look at my assets and liabilities. I think my assets were in the here and now, and my liabilities were in the past.

When I looked back true my life I could see my personality flaws and graces. I could also see my defects of character and how destructive they had been for me and others in my life.

I saw it necessary for me to accept all the positive gifts of thought that I was receiving with a deep humility and understanding.

At the end of the day we can only be worth as much as our souls are worth.

Secretly I wished God had a complaint board or an Ombudsman, and I could stand there and tell them there wrong, they picked the wrong man for can- sir.

God knows the aches and pains of all our hearts.
Gods mercy and love for us can break down the temple of hardness in our cold own hearts.

I believe the Holy Spirit has the power to soften the most hardened of hearts.
God created us in our mother's womb and he alone determines the day of our death.

No human can or should predict this day.
For if he does he takes on and challenges Gods will.

We all must be ready to hand over the full weight of our sufferings, and we must not take them back, otherwise we are back to where we started.

All this stuff going on in my head really felt like spiritual rehabilitation.
I realise now that none of us will ever be perfect, and at times we will disappoint ourselves and others.

To me now the word ego means (edge God out.)
We must give our selves the opportunity to change the things in our life's that don't work, for if we keep doing the same things and expect different results that proves we are truly insane.

We must focus on the problem of life rather than dwelling on the solution.
If we don't make a decision to turn our lives over to God every day, we may become overwhelmed with our fear of life, and our faith will gradually disappear from our minds.

When this can- sir episode began I had no idea that this journey was awaking my sleeping spirit.

We will all face good days and bad days, but we don't have to run from the feelings they produce, we just have to accept them as they are, and let the bad feelings be diminished by the good ones.

Slowly and surely my thoughts were being guided towards a spiritual realm, and this realm I feel was lying just below the level of my consciousness.

As time went by I found it easier to tap into those spiritual resources at my disposal.

As I sat on the train I found myself giving thanks to God for all the things that had gone well for me in my life.

I felt as long as I faced each day that I had left with gratitude, grace and respect, and honesty all would be well.

I realised now that humble people are so close to the ground it's very hard for them to fall, and Self-righteous and arrogant people are so high up in the clouds, that when they fall they will probably damage their spirit.

The Holy Spirit is truly our greatest gift of all; it has the power to guide and shape and sharpens our lives.

I have learned very quickly that when I hold on to grievances, the only one that really suffers is my self.

All too often in my life I cut my nose off despite my face, and I misdirected the energy that I needed to have a more positive and meaningful life.

I feel that all the grievances in my life had led me to a restless spirit within, and this was one of the factors that led to my can- sir.

From That day on my confidence in Gods love was my crutch and my deepest resources.

I think that a vital step in healing is to love our selves, love our enemies, and cherish our true friends.

We humans seem to complicate things.

It was Albert Einstein who said, "Things should be made as easy as possible, but no simpler."

One of Judge Judy's famous statements is,

"Keep it simple, stupid." That statement sums a lot up for me.

All my life I complicated things, and I turned difficulties into disasters.

Now I feel the tide is turning.

I am learning to turn disasters into every day difficulties of life.

Now I am starting to laugh at who I used to be, and I am sorry to me, for having a closed mind for most of my life.

As the train chugged on, I felt like I was receiving spiritual blessings and graces.

These blessings were infusing me with a sense of joy and liberation.

Till this moment I had built up a lot of negative thoughts feelings and emotions about can- sir, which had the capability to destroy and distort my mind and body.

I felt like my natural world and the spiritual world were starting to intertwine. As I sat there I was counting my blessings. This was something I didn't do often enough in my life.

I wondered how many people stop counting their blessings as the weight of life bears down on their shoulders.

The dark clouds were disappearing from the deepest recesses of my mind, and I got a great sense that the days ahead would be days of freedom and liberation.

From deep within my heart and mind I thanked and praised the unseen god of my understanding.

I thanked the all powerful father of the universe for bringing me this far, and I asked for guidance to break the bonds of death if it be his will.

I was learning to absorb and tolerate an enormous amount of stress and pressure.

By now I realise I was on an inward journey to find out what makes me tic, and what keeps me going and energises me when the chips are down.

I don't think up to this point I lived a well balanced and integrated life.

I think over the last ten years I lost the sense and purpose and meaning, and balance of life.

I had lost the sense of being well.

I always felt like I was under a lot of stress and pressure from my self and others. All this pressure continued to build up until it eventually it began to cause me harm.

Not just physical, harm it also caused me a lot of psychological and spiritual damage.

As a child I picked up a lot of negative vibes and messages, and stored them in the hard drive of my brain.

I think this moulded my life, and life style.

Once I understood these things about my self, I felt like I was being released from the grip of the worst winter that the planet has ever endured.

All my life it felt like I was on the road to nowhere.

Now I felt I was on a motorway to redemption, and on all the directional signs they read S.O.S save our souls.

I was feeling the need to be enlightened and sustained in the arms of God.

I was joining my self with my suffering, and this was leading me to a peaceful state of mind body and soul.

I was learning to harness the gifts within my heart and soul. This gave me a very nurturing feeling in every single cell in my body.

I found it amassing that in spite of all my faults and silly little defects, the spiritual world was awakening within me.

I felt like I was one of Gods lost sons, and he sent out the Holy Spirit to find me and help me and heal me.

It became clear to me that most of my life I made my own misery and I am one hundred percent certain that God would like to see me happy and full of life again.

I wondered did I set out to make myself sick. If I did I was surely going to find a way to make myself well again.

The train was reaching the end of its journey

I was starting to feel a bit down hearted and confused.

I was angry with God and I gave him a mouthful from within my mind.

Here I was suddenly blaming others and God for my can- sir, and I was a master at excusing myself.

The reality was I was doing an internal investigation on myself in the privacy of my mind and soul.

I wanted to know what this life was all about.

I wondered was there truly a universal system of justice love, and most of all in my case compassion.

Simply just wishing for the best was not good enough for me.

I know now that the effort and investment I make to survive will be equal to the outcome of my pending surgeries with the help of God and his blessed Mother.

The strange thing is I felt healthy and well in the body before I found out I had can- sir, and my life was pretty stable and easy going.

I thought to myself I had this can- sir for a while without knowing could I have the power to heal it without knowing. Or could the god of my understanding cure me and give me a more meaningful life.

All my life I felt I was searching for something.

Now it was all right to stop searching because I think I found something that can't be list, and that something was my faith and trust in God.

I was slowly making spiritual progress and internal growth was flourishing and abundant within me.

All these spiritual opportunities and in-depth insights were like mini miracles to me.

This was the first time in my life that I was giving my self the opportunity to truly love my self.

I believe everyone should have the opportunity to love themselves on a deeper level than the human level.

Here I was steaming towards Dublin and I felt like I was under god's umbrella.

It seemed like the higher my hope in God was the more gifts I was receiving.

I think I was being empowered to be better and do better.

All my life I complained to myself that no body understood me. I didn't understand myself, how in the name of God did I expect others to understand me.

I realised now that all the sorrow I injured through my life was God's gift to exercise my mind.

I understood now that the things of the earth are no good for my soul.

My soul was thirsty for all the things that are divine and nourishing to my inner self.

My faith was starting to ignite the depths of my soul and spirit.

Most of my life I plunged myself into the satisfaction of self will. Now I found myself plunging in at the deep end of Gods will.

It was obvious to me and to others I was undergoing a serious shifting in my way of thinking.

It was a bit overwhelming.

I knew that the best thing that I could do was to focus on the positive, and to offer God thanks for my life.

I briefly closed my eyes and I wished I had Gods phone number because I had a million and one questions to ask him, and these questions were straight from my heart and soul.

As I closed my eyes I asked God and his holy spirit to help me choose what is right, and help me reject what is wrong.

I asked God for patience peace and self control.

I wondered was I going to survive here on earth, or was I going to be shifted to the heavens above.

I thought either way if I leave this world I would get to see my two children that Mary and I lost two years ago.

If I survived I could stay here and cherish the children that I have.

Thank God I was attaining the ability to look deep within my self and in doing so; I was giving my self the chance to observe and learn, and maybe the chance to heal from deep within.

My body soul and mind was preparing me for all eventualities even death.

I had to keep attention and focus on the surgeries ahead of me, and I had to persevere even when everything seemed hopeless and pointless.

I feel like God was using my pending death to teach me the value and importance of a meaningful life.

There were no certainties for the road ahead of me just a path to follow, and I had to adapt and change as the journey through can- sir progressed.

There were a lot of good feelings and thoughts coming out of my difficulties, and these were fuelling me with the ability and confidence to overcome whatever obstacles I was to face on my journey through and beyond can- sir.

Here I was in the middle of the biggest crisis in my life and I found myself, or should I say God maintaining a good humour within my heart and soul and mind.

I found myself asking my creator to go easy on my physical suffering, and would he help me to fight a good fight.

After all he and he alone knows what's best for me and his will be done regardless of my will.

I was driving out the sad feelings and starting to enjoy the good ones.

I was also starting to accept the highs and lows along the road of can- sir.

I felt emancipated from the past, and now my thoughts were free to accept and believe things in a different way a spiritual way.

I was carefully studying the path I was on, and I had a lot of obstacles in my way. I thought if I can't get through these obstacles I will jump over them, and if they are too high, I will dig under them, and if I can't dig under them then I would just have to blast my way through them, either way my heart was fuelled and filled with determination to face the challenges ahead.

I was trying to figure out what weapons I needed with me in this battle of the mind body and soul.

For my mind I needed faith.

For my body I needed strength.

And for my soul I needed love.

These were three weapons that I could totally rely on.

I was enlarging the power of my soul by accepting my suffering and uniting them with God.

I was surrendering myself to the Devine and precious light.

In doing so I was allowing Gods gifts and powers, and graces to reveal themselves to me.

By now I was adapting to the circumstances of my ill health, and I accept without moan or groan that this was the path chosen for me, and not by me.

I looked at the challenges ahead for me as an opportunity to transform or transcend myself into who I should have being or who God wants me to be.

I understood that day on the train that if God is with me together we can be a devastating force of light and love that no power on earth can stop destroy or change.

Chapter Eight:
Dublin

The train pulled in at Connelly station and came to a sudden stop. I wished the train journey would go on for longer, but that was the old enemy fear creeping back into my mind.

Mary and I stepped of the train. I carried our bags to a taxi and popped them in the boot.

Fifteen minutes later we were at the hotel that Theresa my angel in Boulder city had booked for us.

All of a sudden I remembered I was supposed to ring the hospital at eight o clock that morning for confirmation of an available bed.

Straight away Mary got on her cell phone and rang the hospitals admissions office and asked the girl, "Was there a bed available."

To my horror there was not.

Deep inside me I was fretting, and I wondered now would one day make a difference.

Mary knew by the look on my face that I was stuck in a bit of internal turmoil.

Mary said, "Shit Tony cop on its all ok they want you in the hospital at eight o clock in the morning."

I told Mary I was going to starve to death if I didn't get something to eat.

Than Mary told me that they told her that I can eat all day long if I wanted to, but I would have to start fasting at twelve that night.

We went to the lobby of the hotel and checked in.

To my surprise the woman behind the counter passed me two envelopes and said, "Tony these are for you."

I looked at the envelopes they had American stamps on them.

I opened the first one and it was a get well soon card signed by most of P.C. employees, this immensely lifted my spirit.

I opened the second letter and there was a small note which read;

"Tony you are probably the strongest will person that I have known. Hang in there and be strong because we have unfinished business, As soon as you get well, get your ass back over here and you can look after me for a while."

I thought if this man believes in the strength in me, I better believe in me.

There was also a check in that envelope for two thousand American dollars with no explanation for what it was for.

Mary and I went up to the hotel room and laid our bags on the beds.

I picked up the phone and asked for an outside line and immediately I was given one.

Mary said, "What are you doing."

I replied I am ringing P.C.

Mary said, "It's nearly midnight in Boulder city it's to late you will wake P.C. up. Leave it till about eleven o clock tonight."

Now I had the rest of the day to kill time maybe kill time is not the right words it sounds so morbid.

Mary and I got spruced up and headed out for a big slap up meal.

We walked across O Connell bridge and around the city until we came across Star Bucks coffee house.

I was thrilled to bits because this was my favourite coffee in the whole world, and here it was on sale in Ireland.

I got the coffee and we sat outside and smoked a couple of cigarettes.

I sat and watched the countless people go by, and I wondered are they all well and healthy and free from can- sir.

I wondered would the world ever get their act together in relation to can- sir, and if not, I felt can- sir would destroy countless generations to come.

My tummy was rumbling again it was telling me its time for a big slap up meal.

From where I was sitting I could see a busy Italian restaurant straight across the road.

We both decided to eat there.

As we crossed the road a speeding car flew past the two of us, and came close to knocking us down.

This incident scared the living day lights out of us.

My journey could have finished there and than.

Thank God and his blessed mother it didn't end.

We got two nice window seats in the restaurant and we ordered our meal. I ordered a twelve ounce steak and chips topped off with a salad, and Mary ordered just salad and garlic bread and olives.

This was the best steak I had ever had its amazing how wonderful something tastes when you think its going to possibly be your last.

We finished our meal and Mary decided in order to take my mind off things, we would go shopping.

I agreed and off we went.

I really had no interest but I went any way.

As we shopped my mind was not really with me.

I was fearful for what was before me.

I thought to myself, had I lowered the odds of survival by putting off surgery for a week.

I wondered had I upset Gods rhythm of things, and was he angry with me.

At that very moment I wanted to cry bitterly for what had become of my life. I was struggling to avoid shedding tears. I was afraid that if I started crying I would find it very hard to stop.

The centre of Dublin was not the right place for a grown man to break down and cry.

With all my strength of will I bravely held back the tears within my poor broken mind.

Mary could see that I was in a state of high anxiety and tension.

She asked me to go back to the hotel and watch television and relax. I agreed and she gave me her shopping bags and off I went.

Chapter Nine:
Strange Church

I was walking towards Saint Stephens's green where I came across a small church just off a main street.

I felt compelled to enter.

I sat down at the back of the church and I began to pray.

Here I was bearing my soul to the God of my understanding.

I was confiding in the lord of heaven and Earth.

I asked to be given strength of mind and body, and could I have some peace and joy.

As I lifted my head suddenly out of nowhere there was an old woman sitting in front of me. She turned her head and looked at me. She gave me the biggest smile a human can give. As I smiled back I felt a rush of comfort through all my body from the tips of my hair to the nails on my toes.

I sensed a fabulous ghostly presence from this old lady.

I bowed my head to continue to pray. I wondered who was this woman, and how in the name of God was I feeling an uplifted soul from deep within.

I walked to the alter of the church, and knelt down and asked God to be with me, as I journeyed towards my possible earthly doom.

I prayed for God and his Saints, and his Angels to be with me through my possible fleeting hours of life.

I got up off my knees and walked out the side door of the church.

I put my hand in the font of holy water and I blessed my self.

As I stepped out the old lady was there partially blocking my way.

She smiled again at me and straight away she asked me for some change.

I smiled back and pulled a couple of euro out of my pocket and gave it to her.

She thanked me and asked me my name.

I told her my name is Tony.

She said, "No no your full name."

I told her my full name was Anthony Thomas Power.

She paused for a brief moment and said, "That's a powerful name."

I replied, what do you mean by that?

She said, "Did you know Saint Anthony is the saint of lost things, and you should be honoured to bear his name." I was a bit freaked out by now.

This old lady said, "Its not only things that Saint Anthony finds for people, he also finds damaged souls and hands them over to God for repair."

I was a bit stunned and taken back by what she was saying.

She said that Thomas was special in the eyes of God, and I was to bear his name with honour and pride.

She told me to stop doubting the wonderful things that were happening.

Then out of the blue she said, "You will be all right your can- sir will be sorted out from the heavens above."

When she mentioned the word can- sir I nearly jumped out of my skin.

In my conversation with this old lady I didn't mention can- sir but she knew, and I was dumb struck.

As I left the church behind that day my head was amazed and amused and bewildered.

I wondered how she knew of my illness.

I thought did she smell it coming from me, or did she know by the look on my face, or did she somehow over hear my prayers while I was in the church.

I being the doubter in my rational mind, I thought to myself, is this random guess for some spare change.

In my spiritual world it seemed like this lady was there to comfort and reassures me that all would be well.

I slowly walked back to the hotel.

When I got there I went straight to the bar, and ordered a pint of Guinness and pumped it down my throat.

I was feeling a bit drunk, so I went straight to the room and lay on the bed.

It was five thirty in the evening, and there was no sign of Mary.

I phoned her cell phone and she answered, and told me she would be at least an hour if not more.

I was dizzy from the Guinness so I took my shoes off and knelt down beside the bed and grabbed my Rosary Beads from my pocket and I began to pray. I said the full Rosary and when I was finished I lay down on the bed.

As I lay there in silence and peace, my thought deepened.

It began to dawn on me that there was more to can- sir then just the physical stuff.

I could feel that there was psychological and spiritual stuff to deal with; all in one big package called can- sir.

I owned this package, God had addressed it to me, it was mine and mine alone.

That evening I understood that God wanted me to survive and there were three things I would have to do for him.

One was to change everything I do.

Two was to change everything I think.

Three was to change everything I say.

I was slowly attaining the ability to be open minded, and I was willing to accept the crosses that were bestowed on me.

I understood that if I wanted to try and understand God, I would have to try and understand myself first.

In some strange way all my internal dialog was broadening and deepening my sense of faith and courage.

All these thoughts gave me a sense of unity, unity with God as I understood him.

I understood that if God is with me who or what can be against me.

As I lay there I felt comforted and consoled from a place beyond human comprehension.

I embraced these feelings and stored them in my brain, so I could recall them in times of desperation and need.

Suddenly there was a knock on the door I was startled. I arose sharply and answered the door.

It was Mary and both her hands were full and laidened down with shopping bags.

Mary asked me, how was my evening?

I told her I that on my way back to the hotel, I went into a church.

I told Mary about the old lady and what she said.

I didn't know whether she would believe me or not, so I told her any way. She was amazed and amused, but she didn't doubt me. She encouraged me to believe this old lady rather than doubt the old lady.

Mary asked me was I drinking. I guess she could smell it from my breath.

I said yes I had a pint of Guinness to settle my nerves.

By now I was hungry again and Mary asked me would I like something to eat.

I said yes, but I don't want to go out.

Mary suggested that we get a take away, and asked would I like fish and chips or pizza.

I replied fish and chips please.

Right she said "I passed a nice smelling fish and chip shop a block or so away from here."

Mary said, "I will go and get the food, and you wait here, I will be back in fifteen minutes."

Mary left the hotel room and I lay back on the bed.

As I lay there my thought deepened. I wondered was I walking into possible doom, and was this up coming event the end of my days on this planet.

I asked myself were these the fleeting hours of life?

The human side of me was scared and in shock.

The new found spiritual side of me was infused and invigorated with the thoughts of heaven and heavenly things.

There and then I asked God for the strength and wisdom.

That I may stand my ground and not give way under the pressure of can-sir.

I was feeling a sense of inward liberty and inward love for myself. This was a new feeling for me. All my life I never felt this liberty and love.

I solemnly swore to my self to keep fear out of the equation, for now I knew that fear would have a controlling influence over me and my mind and my

Can-sir.

I picked up my Rosary Beads from the pillow and knelt down on the floor beside the bed.

I remember so well that every decade was for other people in my life.

One decade was for my children, Elaine and Shane.

The second one was for Mary and her three children.

The third decade was for my mum and dad.

The fourth was for my four brothers and two sisters.

The fifth was for all the people's souls that had died from can-sir.

Mary returned with the fish and chips and a bottle of red wine. We sat on the bed and nibbled away at the food.

Mary popped the wine open and poured two glasses.

She handed me a glass, and in one slug the glass was empty.

I asked for another one and was told no, so I left it at that.

We finished our food and Mary drank what was left of the wine.

I switched the television on for Mary, I tried to settle and focus on it myself.

I was wasting my time for my mind was in a different place all together.

I desperately needed some fresh air.

I asked Mary did she want to come with me, "Where?" she said. I replied for a walk and a few cigarettes.

Her answer was no, she said she was too tired and the shopping took all her energy. I didn't doubt her.

I said ok than, I will see you in a while.

I left the room and went to the hotel smoking area just outside the main door and sat down.

I lit my cigarette and tried to relax my conscious mind, but it was impossible. I felt like my poor brain was travelling at a million miles a second heading for outer space.

I sat there wondering what to do.

I realised no matter what I think do or say, my future has already being decided by God.

I wondered was I going to the land of the Gods, or was I staying in the land of humans.

I pulled my Rosary beads from my pocket and held them tightly in my hand; this gave me a sense of comfort and trust and peace.

I wondered what I should or shouldn't be doing to help myself through and beyond can- sir.

As I lit my second cigarette I understood deep in my mind to assume the best in order to achieve the best.

I prayed to God and the Queen of the universe for the willingness to broaden and open my narrow mind.

There is no doubt about it my human side was scared.

On the other hand my spiritual side was being strengthened by my prayers meditation, and actions and thoughts.

I realised that wishing and dreaming was part of my will, and not Gods will for me.

I couldn't fool myself any more.

That night the whole of me accepted that I had a progressive and fatal disease.

I could spend all my precious time arguing in my head for things to turn out my way, which never really worked anyway.

On the other hand I could surrender my will to the God of my understanding, and wait for peace and happiness to flow.

I felt a sense of peace in my soul, and I think this was due to the fact that I was accepting the ebb and flow of my life.

I wondered did God put me in this awkward position in order to be closer to him, in my hours of desperate need.

I really think the answer was yes.

All my life I thought it was other peoples fault.

Now I was doing an internal investigation of my life in the privacy of my own heart and mind.

I could see a lot of stubbornness in my past, and I suppose this got me into trouble with others all my life.

Chapter Ten:
The Night and Morning
of My First Surgery

I looked at my watch it was nine o clock and I had eleven hours to go for my trip to the Mater Hospital.

It seemed like I was getting ready to go into battle; a battle of fear and fearlessness all wrapped in one big bundle, just for me and me alone.

I felt like my soul was under a regime of rehabilitation and rejuvenation, and my faith was stronger than my fear. I was learning to be content no matter what state I was in.

I put my precious Rosary Beads back in my pocket and I went back into the hotel.

I let myself into the room with the swipe card.

Mary was watching the news on the television.

Suddenly the phone in the room rang Mary said, "Pick it up." I did and it was my old friend Paul. C. Fisher.

I could hear in his voice that he was happy to hear me.

I told him all about my journey home.

He told me that all along he felt I was different, and that he had never met anybody as straight and as truthful as me. He asked me was there anything that I wanted or needed.

I said, no Paul all as I need is some prayers from you and the gang over there.

He said, "Consider it done."

Paul said, "Tony you are a survivor, and I could see it in your eyes while you were here."

He said, "The God in you is willing you to live don't let him down be strong and be true to yourself."

I asked him how he was keeping, he said, "fine and by the way Tony I found the secret to life."

I wondered what in the name of God he was babbling on about.

Then he said to me, "Tony the secret is to keep breathing no matter what happens in life."

I found this so funny but simple and true, coming from a healthy man ninety two years of age. Paul wished me well and said, "Can you put Mary on the phone."

I handed the phone to Mary and they spoke to each other for a good fifteen minutes. Mary hung up the phone and as soon as she did it rang again.

She picked it up immediately. It was her mum in Los Angeles.

They spoke for a few minutes and Mary handed me the phone.

I was so genuinely happy to hear her voice.

She asked me how things were going there.

I told her I was hanging in there, and I felt I was getting stronger by the minute.

She replied, "Tony I hope you are still pouring the blood of Jesus Christ over your kidneys." I said no but; as soon as I get of the phone I will do it.

She told me to get a pen and some paper and write this down. So I did and this is the way it goes.

Throughout my busy, bustling day,
Someone waits for me.

A dozen things I've yet to do,
Still someone waits for me.

And when my day is finally done
In a moment of solitude I learn,

That god has being here all day long,
Patiently waiting for my return.

God's gentle presence fills my heart,
My thoughts are calmed, my mind at rest.

God lets me know that all is well,
And gives me strength for any test.

So I will start out each new day,
With God's love assuring me,

That no matter what it holds,
Someone always waits for me.

We spoke for at least another fifteen minutes.

Out of the blue she told me she had can- sir- twice in her life.

I was more than surprised for this was the first person that I could truly identify with.

She said, "Tony don't leave anybody steal your light."

She wished me success on my journey and said, "May God be with your every breath."

I said god bless you, and hung up the phone.

I lay on the bed and I wished these dark days would be over.

At this stage I realised that it takes insight and courage in order to take personal responsibility for my life and my can- sir.

I looked over at Mary she was nodding off to sleep.

I thought it best not to disturb her, for her day was as long as mine, if not longer.

I lay there thinking about the range of emotions and feeling that can- sir had brought to my mind and to my life.

The bad feelings were shock, disbelief, anger, fear and sadness.

The good feelings were hope, courage, faith, wisdom and insight.

I was tired and I could not switch off the washing machine effect of my thoughts.

My thoughts were like a lucky dip, you don't know what's going to come out next.

By now Mary's breathing had elevated to a snore, she was fast asleep.

I set the alarm for six in the morning.

I also rang the hotel reception and asked for a wake up call for six fifteen in the morning.

I opened my hospital bag and took out my new funky biker mice P.Jays.

I put them on, and in the dim lit room I looked at the mirror. I really looked like an adult dressed like a child ready for bed.

This made me laugh at myself.

I thought to myself if this is my last night on the Earth and I go to God tomorrow, he will have a good giggle at my funky P.Jays.

I lay back on the bed and, I clutched my Rosary Beads and began to pray the Rosary.

As I was praying my mind was drifting to places of peace and comfort that I had being in my life.

I found myself in my mind, in Mount Mellary praying at the grotto to the queen of the universe.

By now my prayers were not asking for anything. I was offering my prayers as a way of saying thank you to God and his angels for all that has being, for all that is, and for all that is to come.

I must have drifted into a deep sleep.

I suddenly woke up, I looked at the clock it was three in the morning and I felt strangely fresh and in possession of all my senses.

I sensed a gentle presence in the room and the hair on my arms and the back of my neck instantly stood up.

I got out of bed and went for a pe pe.

I got back into bed and lay there wondering what I was feeling in the room.

I became conscious of my breathing and my heart beat.

They were both in a heightened state.

Even though I was lying on the bed I felt elevated from the bed, I kind of felt weightless.

I had no blankets on top of me, but yet I still felt covered.

This covering felt like I was wrapped in a cloak from head to toe.

I wondered was this some sort of spiritual protection.

Was this the cloak of our lady protecting me for the journey ahead? Or was I losing the plot and going insane.

I continued giving thanks through my prayers, and I guess I must have drifted off to sleep again.

Suddenly the alarm went off, I lay there and I did not want to turn it off.

Some how in my silly mind I wanted to freeze time.

I suppose this was my human fear creeping back in.

Mary reached over and turned the alarm clock off.

I got out of bed and put the coffee on the boil.

Mary went and had a shower.

I sat there watching the coffee boil and I wondered was this going to be my last coffee.

Mary finished her shower, and I popped in there, and scrubbed myself from head to toe.

As I washed I wondered was this my last wash while on this planet.

As I stood there tears streamed down my face.

I remember them so well, they were tears of fear, and they were tears of anger, all in one package just for me and me alone.

I finished my shower and put my biker mice P.Jays back on. I sat down with Mary and we had our coffee.

When we finished the coffee Mary said, "Put your clothes on, we are walking to the hospital, both of us need the fresh air." And for humour she said,

"If you're a good boy I will get you a star buck's coffee on the way."

To me this was the best incentive any one could give me to get me moving.

I agreed and I pulled a tracksuit bottoms over my P.Jays and put my new granddad cardigan on.

It was seven A.M. and Mary said, "For the love of god will you hurry up your like a little old lady rushing around and getting nothing done."

Mary knelt down by one of the beds and put her hand under. She pulled out a large plastic bag and said, "This is for you Tony."

I opened the bag and to my surprise it was a large white polar bear teddy.

Mary said, "You better give him a name before he goes to the hospital with you."

Without even thinking the name Kidney popped into my mind.

I told Mary his name and she burst into an uncontrollable laugh.

She found it extremely funny and so did I.

But that was his name and under no circumstances was I going to change it.

For some strange reason I felt Kidney was going to be with me in my darkest hours and he was and still is.

I had an instant wonderful child like affection for kidney.

He was like my gushy baby blanket.

I could hold on to him tightly come hell or high water.

Mary said, "Hurry up Tony stick your stuff in your bag and don't forget your tooth brush."

I quickly packed the last few bits and pieces and I was ready for my first journey through and beyond hospital.

We left the hotel room and went outside to the smoking area. We sat down and smoked a cigarette.

When we were finished Mary said, "Put kidney in your bag." I said why?

She said, "You're going to look like a fool carrying a toy polar bear through the streets of Dublin."

I said, I know but I just don't care.

I straddled kidney over the top of my bag and I wheeled him behind me.

I said to Mary that I wanted to go to the church that I was in yesterday.

Mary agreed and said, "We will be late but I suppose it doesn't really matter."

I brought Mary the same way as I walked yesterday.

We walked for about twenty minutes and to my amazement I could not find the small church that I was in yesterday.

I was one hundred percent sure I was on the same street as yesterday.

I asked two people did they know of a small church near by.

They both said, "There is no church around here."

Mary looked at me in a bewildering way and said, "I hope you're not losing the plot Tony."

Mary said, "Were you day dreaming or did you imagine this."

I was gob smacked and I had no answer for Mary.

As a matter of fact my gob has never being so smacked.

By now my brain was very muddled and confused.

I could not understand this event.

As we walked on I wondered was I going mad, was I losing the plot, or had my brain being tampered with from the heavens above.

I was confused and totally restless in my mind.

I looked at my watch it was seven forty five as we reached Star Buck's coffee house.

I ordered Mary a cappuccino and the strongest coffee that they had, with an extra shot of coffee in it for me.

We sat outside and sipped our coffee and smoked a cigarette.

I sat there motionless and I thought to my self I have two choices here one is to stand firm and fight.

Two is to pick up my bag and take flight and high tail it out of here as soon as possible.

It felt harder to choose the first option but thank God and his blessed mother I did.

We picked up our coffee and began to walk towards the Mater hospital, as I walked my whole body was trembling with fear; my legs were unsteady as I walked on.

My hands were shaking as I spilled what coffee I had left.

A hundred meters or so in the distance, I could see the Mater hospital.

Part of it was very old and gothic looking, and part of it was very modern looking.

Straight across the road from the old part of the hospital I could see a church. We walked up to it.

I said to Mary I got to go in here for a few minutes.

Mary said, "Do you realise it's nearly half past eight and you are late."

Ok I said just give me five minutes and we will go into the hospital.

I knelt down by a statue of the queen of the universe and began to pray and ask for guidance and courage for the future if there was one for me.

Chapter Eleven:
Entering the Hospital

I finished my prayers and we left the church, and went straight across the road and entered the hospital.

Instinctually I went straight to a coffee machine just inside the door of the hospital and got some coffee for Mary and me.

Mary took my coffee and said, "Are you mad, you're supposed to be fasting."

I suppose in the madness and panic and turmoil of it all, I genuinely forgot that I was supposed to be fasting

We went outside the main door and Mary had her coffee and we smoked a cigarette.

I sucked the cigarette in to me. I suppose my nerves were at there wits end. I smoked it like it was the last cigarette on Earth.

Mary finished her cigarette, and we went back into the hospital.

We went straight to the admittance office reception and took a ticket and waited. To my amazement my number was one hundred and seventeen.

We sat down, my two knees were knocking together and my heart was pounding violently.

Mary put her hand on my knee and told me to calm down.

I took a deep breath and calmed down.

Suddenly my ticket number appeared on a L.E.D. screen.

We got up and entered the office.

Mary and I sat down and the lady there asked me for all my details.

I answered all her questions, then she pushed a few buttons on a strange looking machine, and a hospital identity wrist band popped out of the machine.

She told me to go straight to Saint Anthony's ward.

She gave me a small map of the hospital and we left her office.

Without even speaking to Mary, we wandered out the main entrance to the smoking area and lit up our cigarettes.

We finished our smoke and went back into the hospital.

Mary had the map so she led the way to the ward.

As we walked down a very long corridor I noticed it was all painted green.

I wondered to my self was this my personal green mile.

Its scary the way the head thinks when one is facing imminent danger or the threat of death.

We arrived at the ward and entered.

I scanned the whole ward within five seconds.

There were eight beds there and a small nurse's station off to the right with a big observation window overlooking the ward.

The sister of the ward approached us and in a kind gentle voice said, "Can I help ye."

I said yes as I showed her my wrist band.

She briefly read it, and directed me to my bed.

To my surprise the number of the bed was one.

I felt a small bit of comfort in feeling I was in the right place, bed number one in Saint Anthony's ward.

The sister told me to put my P.Jays on and get into bed.

I slipped my runners and track suit off and sat up on the bed.

The sister looked at me with a bright smile on her face and said, "Tony they are the coolest P.Jays I've ever seen in my life."

I reached over the side of the bed and picked Kidney from the top of my bag, and put him on the bed beside me.

The ward sister looked at me with a slight grin on her face and said, "Your teddy is gorgeous, has he a name."

Yes I said I named him Kidney.

The sister suddenly broke into a fit of laughter.

When she stopped she said, "Tony I can see were going to have a ball of a time while you're here."

She said to me, "Lie back and relax, and the team of surgeons will be along in a half hour or so."

Mary left the ward to go for a smoke, and I lay down on the bed.

I raised my eyes and to my surprise I could see out the window on the opposite side of the ward, the church that I had being in earlier that morning.

I felt a sense of comfort being so close to God's house.

Over the next ten minutes or so I must have gazed at the church at least twenty times, and each time my levels of stress were slowly diminishing.

Mary returned and sat down on the chair beside me, and asked me did the surgeons come yet.

Just as the words came out of Mary's mouth the team of surgeons entered the ward and came directly over to me.

The junior surgeon Mister Murphy said to me, "Tony we are going to run some tests on your heart, and if all is well we will proceed with the surgery shortly after lunch."

I said no problem Mister Murphy that suits me fine.

"O by the way he said nice teddy bear."

I said its not a teddy bear, it's a polar bear and his name is Kidney.

The two surgeons and the two nurses with them burst out laughing. I guess they found this very funny due to their profession.

Mister Murphy asked me had I any questions.

I said yes he said, "Fire away."

I asked him how many of this type of surgeries had he done.

He replied, "Roughly about one hundred."

I replied and said will you do me one big favour. He said, "What's that."

I said will you try make this one the pinnacle of your career.

He grabbed my hand and held it tightly, and put his mouth close to my ear, and in a soft gentle voice said, "Stop worrying, you're so lucky to have me, I am the best there is, and I am not going to let any thing happen to a man from my own county."

He said, "Tony it would be advisable to take something to relax."

There was no hesitation from me, yes was my answer.

He asked the nurse to give me five mill grams of Diazepam, she did and within five to ten minutes I was feeling drowsy and totally relaxed.

I suppose within ten to fifteen minutes the porter arrived with a wheel chair. He was full of humour he said, "Get in mister power were going joy riding."

I got in and off we went to the cardiac unit for my tests.

The tests lasted a half an hour, and the doctor their told me that my heart was one hundred and ten percent.

The porter wheeled me back to Saint Anthony's ward, and I got back into the bed.

As I lay there I was thrilled to bits to think that God had given me a good strong heart.

Suddenly my cell phone rang. It was Mary she had slipped out for breakfast. Mary asked me did I want or need any thing.

I replied no I am fine for every thing, thank you.

Mary said, "See you in ten minutes."

The ward sister and two Pilipino nurses came over to me.

The sister did my bloods and one of the nurses puffed up my pillows for me.

The sister said, " Tony the bloods will be back in an hour, and if all is well the surgeons will go ahead with your surgery straight after lunch."

Mary returned and sat on the bed and held my hand and said nothing.

Somehow I could sense her fear for me.

I told Mary that the heart test was fine, and I am waiting on the results of the bloods.

I could smell smoke on Mary's clothes, and the craving for a cigarette became the only thing on my mind at that present moment.

I called the ward sister over and asked her could I go out for a cigarette. To my surprise she said, "If it works Tony go for it."

I was thrilled to bits.

Mary and I bolted for the main door at the old part of the hospital. We sat on the steps and smoked our cigarettes.

We talked for a short time, and finally we went back to the ward.

As I got back into the bed, I wondered how long I was going to be here in this bed.

Tension and worry was starting to creep back into my mind.

I was burning out on the inside, and I tried not to show it on the outside.

As I struggled with my thoughts. I wondered could God give me a predated ticket into Heaven or could he at least delay my entry for a few years.

It's just as well I wasn't thinking out loud because everybody in Saint Anthony's ward would have questioned my sanity.

I was overwhelmed with the fear of death.

At this stage I wished I had my own internal sleeping potion that I could switch on right now, and switch it off again sometime in the future.

Suddenly a porter walked in to the ward and handed some paper work to the sister. I guessed it was the results of the bloods.

The sister walked over to my bed and put the paper work on the clip board at the end of the bed.

My guess was right it was my blood results.

The sister said, "Tony your bloods are perfect, and were going ahead with your surgery in about an hour or so." She also gave me a surgical gown a pair of stockings and a hat to put on. She then disappeared into the observation room of the ward.

I undressed and I put the gown and hat on.

I lay there thinking of the violence of the process of

Surgery and the physical pain it would bring to me.

I picked my beads up from the top of my locker, and began to silently pray for the physical strength to get through this surgery.

As I lay their, I wondered was my soul pure enough to get me through the pearly gates of Heaven.

I said an act of contrition and asked the God of my understanding to forgive me for all my sins, from the day I was born up till this very moment in time.

Mary reached over and grabbed my hand and said, "Tony snap out of it, you look like your lost in space and time."

I put my beads around my neck and brought myself from my thoughts, into the here and now.

Time was pressing on; the other people in the ward were being served their lunch. It smelled so divine and wholesome.

It's such a horrible feeling looking at other people eating when you know you're not allowed to eat.

It was now two o clock and the ward sister gave me two tablets to take, and she said to me, "The porter is on his way to bring you to theatre."

I lay their motionless and to tell the truth I was scared and afraid and partially s------g my self.

I was starting to feel drowsy from the two tablets, and I started to wander in and out of a mild sleep.

Mary pinched my nose and I sprang to attention.

As I looked to my left side the porter was standing there and he called my name.

I answered it's me.

He said, "Pop your self on the trolley and relax."

I did and off we went Mary was holding my hand tightly as they walked towards the operating theatre.

Within five minutes we were at the door of the pre- op room.

Mary kissed me softly on the lips and whispered the words, "I love you Tony, please be strong and come back to me, I will be here waiting for you."

As the porter pushed me through the doors I thought to myself this is it, the final show down the grand finale of my life.

Mister Murphy came to me and asked me how I was feeling.

I told him I was bricking it. I don't think he understood what I said.

He then said tony, "Your going to have to take the beads of your neck, you can't have surgery with those beads on."

As groggy as I was I said no their not coming of they are staying on come hell or high water. He had a look of shock and bewilderment on his face.

He said, "Sit tight Tony I will try and sort it out."

He disappeared through a side door and returned to me within five minutes.

He told me he had spoken to mister Akiatar, and he insists that it comes off.

I than told mister Murphy that if the beads were to come off my neck, there was no way my surgery was going ahead. Mister Murphy said, "Tony you're an awkward man."

Suddenly the side door opened and Mister Akiatar came over to me with a stern look on his face.

He stared at me and said, "Tony I see we have a bit of a small problem here."

I said it might be a small problem for you sir, but for some strange reason I feel I need them around my neck.

Mister Akiatar stared at me for a few moments with an intense look on his dark face.

Suddenly he said, "The problem is sorted."

I said what do you mean!

He looked at me and said, "Tony your beads are plastic, and we can disinfect them in a solution, but they will be stained a yellowish colour."

I said it doesn't matter as long as they are on my neck.

I truly don't know to this day, why I was so adamant that the beads would remain around my neck.

I took my Rosary Beads off and handed them to the nurse standing beside me. As soon as I took them off I felt spiritually naked. This feeling scared the living day lights out of me.

The nurse returned within a couple of minutes with my yellowish beads and said, "Lift your head up." I lifted my head up and the nurse slipped the beads over my neck.

Instantly that naked feeling disappeared.

Mister Akiatar looked at me and said, "I think you're a bit of an odd ball." I said you're probably right.

Than he said, "Now you're sorted, have you any other issues."

I said no. In a humorous way He said, "Can we get started now."

I replied yes and like Buzz Light year I said to infinity and beyond. Every body there smiled at my comment.

I felt comfortable but nervous.

The nurse there said, "Tony we are going to put you to sleep now."

I said no problem just make sure you give me plenty of what ever it is that knocks me out.

She said, "No problem" as she injected me with the anaesthetic.

The nurse told me to count to ten and I tried.

I guess I only got to about five and that was it lights out for me.

Six hours later I woke up in the recovery room. I was groggy and drowsy. The first thing I did was check were my beads still around my neck, they were. I was well pleased.

My body was as stiff as a poker, and I felt pain all over. My throat was as dry as a thirsty camel. I lay their thinking at least I am still here and still breathing.

I tried to move my legs but they were dead.

I called the nurse over, I asked her for some water she said, "No Tony you will have to wait at least an hour before you can have anything."

I asked her why she said, "There's a possibility you'll get sick." I accepted this and let it go.

As I lay there I was feeling very hot and sweaty I asked the nurse to pull back the covers, she did.

I looked down at my body, and the first thing I saw was a tube coming from my little man leading to a pe bag.

The second thing I saw was the size of the plaster, it ran from my belly button to my back bone.

In the middle of this big plaster there was another tube coming out, and it was leading to a blood drainage bag. For some strange reason, all I saw did not bother me in the least bit.

Suddenly the double doors swung open and Mister Akiatar and Mister Murphy came straight over to me.

Mister Murphy said, "Tony every thing went according to plan, you done very well."

He said, "Have you any questions or worries Tony."

I asked him why I can't move my legs.

He said, "Tony we inserted an epidural in your back for pain, and every thing below that is numbed for the moment."

He asked me was there anything else.

I said I need some water.

He told me that there was a high chance I would vomit, if I put any thing in my stomach for the next few hours.

I said I will take that chance.

He looked at me and said, "You're off your head. I said you're probably right.

He said, "You can have some water on the condition, you sip it slowly."

I said, yes I will.

The nurse gave me a plastic cup of water, and my first sip was like finding a well in the desert.

As I lay there my mind was hyper active but my body was temporally out of action.

I reached to my neck and took my beads off, and squeezed them tightly in my right hand.

I began to pray and give thanks to the God of the universe for letting me stay here for another while.

I felt like I had being touched by a divine hand.

I was trying to focus my mind in the present, in order to focus on my healing.

All my life I felt I was caught within my own anger and unhappiness at life and about life.

Maybe this led me here, I truly don't know.

I understood now that every thought and breath is so precious, and how I think is how I will be.

I was content in knowing that a force beyond my temporal comprehension was helping me on my journey through can- sir.

I think when God created us all he infused a spirit within us.

I think Gods powers are always ready to meet our every day needs, but we must be the channel through which the power of the Holy Spirit flows.

I figured out that the more I turned and tuned into this inner spirit, the less I felt fear and anxiety for my future.

It seamed like my trust in the awareness of God's presence heightened my faith, and gave me a deep understanding that all will be well for me.

As I lay their thanking God for a successful surgery a sense of peace calm and serenity shrouded me, and it seemed like all my cares and fears were being slowly washed away.

I thanked God and his spirits for bringing me through my first major storm in life.

I understand now that the only way to go forward properly in life, is to acknowledge and accept the inward spirit.

I understood that day, that we are all children of God and God is spirit, there for we are all spiritual beings.

I know now that life changes, day by day. You can fight it to no avail. Change is one of the only things that is constant in life.

I also know we all make mistakes but its how we deal with the aftermath is what defines us as human beings.

We all as individuals have to take responsibility for our lives, and the direction in which were heading.

We have to look deep within our souls, and we have to extinguish any bad values that reside there.

I feel there is no currency available on Earth that will get us through the pearly gates of Heaven.

Without a heart and soul we would be just wondering machines, with no purpose or meaning to life.

My time in the recovery room was up.

The nurse there said, "Tony we will bring you back to your ward as soon as we get a porter."

I was thrilled to bits that my first surgery was over and I was still breathing, and I was heading back to Saint Anthony's ward.

The porter arrived and wheeled me out through the double doors. Mary was sitting just outside waiting for me, she grabbed my hand and said, "Thank god and his blessed mother you're alive." I was wheeled back to my ward.

With some difficulty the porter and the two Pilipino nurses slid me back into my bed.

I laid their motionless holding Mary's hand, and I guess I drifted off into a deep sleep.

I woke early the next morning and as soon as I opened my eyes I was in pain it seemed like the epidural was not working properly.

I called the ward sister over to me and told her of my pain.

She gave me two tablets and a glass of water.

I popped them in my mouth, and within ten minutes the pain eased off.

I must have drifted off to sleep again. Suddenly I was woken up, Mary was sitting on the end of the bed we both smiled at each other but we did not speak.

I think the smiles were in recognition of my survival.

Mister Akiatar and Mister Murphy arrived at the ward to do their rounds. Mister Akiatar complimented me on my surgery, and enquired how I was doing. I explained about the pain that I was in. He got a nurse to give me some intravenous morphine.

I said I am in a lot of pain. He said, "You shouldn't be, the epidural in your back should kill the pain."

He said, "If it's not doing its job properly we will take it out."

I could feel the pain slightly dissipating as the seconds passed by. After about five minutes Mister Murphy reached over the bed and gently removed the epidural from my back.

I lay back down and to my surprise the pain was dissipating.

Mister Murphy asked me had I any other problems.

I replied yes, when will you be leaving me home?

He smiled at me and informed me between seven and ten days depending on how well I recovered.

I was thrilled to bits, and I told him I had a goal to aim for.

I also asked him when would the drainage bag on my left side, and the pipe in my little man be removed.

He laughed at me and said, "Maybe tomorrow Tony, it depends on your bloods."

He asked me was I in any discomfort from the tubes.

I said yes my we little man is very raw and sore.

He told the nurse to put some soothing cream on me.

She answered that she would but I said no, no, no, I will do it myself. I guess it must be a man thing.

The surgeons then left the ward.

The nurse gave me the cream, and Mary pulled the curtains over.

I put the cream on and the soreness eased off instantly.

I asked Mary did she have a breakfast, She said, "No Tony." I told her to go and have a good feed.

Suddenly Mary's cell phone rang she answered it, as she left the ward.
She returned within five minutes with a worried look on her face.
I asked her was she ok she replied, and said, "Her mother in law, Florence was on the phone, and the children all came down with some sort of virus.
I told her to get her ass back to Wexford as soon as possible.
Mary said, "What about you." Mary was torn between her worry for me and her worry for the children. I didn't want to add to her burden so I told her not to worry about me because, I am in Gods hands and I feel very well now.
I told Mary to go straight to the hotel and pack her bag and order a taxi straight away. I kissed her as she said, "Are you sure you will be all right."
I kissed her again, and jokingly said, I have Kidney here to keep me company. She smiled at me and told me she loved me.
Look I said I love you too, but for now get your ass to Wexford and sort out the children.
We knew that my mother would be coming some time today.
I think this made her feel at ease about leaving me.
She kissed me and waved goodbye as she left the ward.

As I lay there I was tired, hungry, thirsty, and sore.
I called the nurse over and asked her for something to eat and drink.
She offered me some toast and tea.
She left the ward and within five minutes she returned with the glorious feast.
With a pleasant smile on her pretty young face, she asked me if I would like to sit up. I thought this would be a good idea.
She called the other nurse over and they took an arm each, and pulled me up in the bed.

I began to eat my toast and drink my tea; it was so delicious it tasted like it came straight from heaven.

I finished it in two minutes flat. It was the nicest toast I ever had in my life, even though I don't like toast.

When I was finished I shuffled myself back down in the bed, and snuggled into Kidney and drifted off to sleep.

I was suddenly woken up by a kiss on my cheek.

As I looked up my mum and my son Shane were standing there.

I was over the moon to see them there, and happy to have them beside my bed.

The first thing my mum did was bless me and then she blessed herself, and in a very loud voice she said, "Thank God and his blessed mother you are alright." Even as a grown man my mother could still make a show of me. She can still do it today, maybe it's a gift that all mothers have.

I told her I was still breathing. I looked at Shane and I noticed he had a bewildered look on his face, but I knew he was happy to see me alive. God bless him. I welled up inside and I struggled to hold the tears back. That evening I sensed his worries and fears and it scared the living daylights out of me.

My mum handed me some mass cards and told me that all her friends and acquaintances were praying for me back in Waterford. As soon as she said this I profoundly understood the power of other people's prayers. I felt a sense of hope, because all these other people were out there praying for me to get well again.

My mum sat on the side of the bed and held my hand tightly. As she did this, I was overcome by a sense of comfort and peace. I felt nourished by her touch.

She rubbed my head like one would rub an infants head.

Then suddenly my mums partner Jim appeared.

Jim had come through his own crosses in life, and they were serious ones. He had lost his wife and only son both through illnesses, but you would never think it by the look on his happy go lucky jolly face.

I was happy to see him.

He never spoke much but was always smiling.

I suppose he was happy on the inside.

As I lay there I was happy that Jim was my mum's partner. They were and are still good together; they look after one another as they progress through their later years in life.

My mum explained that they had to get the six o clock train home to Waterford.

I said o- key- do mum I will see you soon. In a drowsy voice, I said thanks for bringing Shane up to see me.

My mum kissed me and said, "Love you Tony," and then she linked Jims arm and left the ward with Shane.

By now I was tired and groggy from the morphine. I needed some sleep.

I switched off my cell phone, and I snuggled my face into Kidney. I drifted off into a deep sleep.

I woke up at about nine that night.

I switched my cell phone on, it started beeping.

I looked at the screen and to my surprise, I had ten missed calls. I was in so much pain that I did not feel anxious or worried about the reasons for all the missed calls.

Straight away I phoned Mary who said she had been ringing me. Because my phone was off she rang the ward. They told her that I was sleeping.

I asked her how the children were. She said, "They are fine they just have a tummy bug."

We chatted for about ten minutes and than we said God bless to each other and hung up.

I turned my head to the left side, and I could see and hear three nurses in the nurses' station sitting and chatting just taking it easy.

As I lay there I mentally assessed my pain level and I guess I scored somewhere between six and eight, ten being the worst.

I was over the moon to be alive, and I was doing my best to be positive and to keep a good spirit within me.

I was ready to go to any lengths to put an end to my disease.

Suddenly from the corner of my left eye I could see one of the pretty Filipino night nurses rising from her chair.

She walked over to my bed and smiled at me. I smiled back.

She plucked my chart from the end of my bed. She briefly looked at it, and then focussed her eyes on the monitors that surrounded me.

She said, "Tony how are you feeling."

I told her that the pain was bearable at the moment.

She than offered me some tea and toast, and without hesitation I answered yes.

She disappeared off the ward and within five minutes returned with the tea and toast for me. She left it on my tray and returned to her station.

I horsed it down, it was delicious.

As I lay their staring at the high ceiling in my ward, my thoughts were beginning to drift to a place of peace and prayer.

This was the first time since my surgery that I had a quiet moment to thank the god of my understanding for our successful surgery.

It felt like my self and my creator had fought the big 'C' and we succeeded for now.

I understood now that dealing with can-sir is the ultimate test of faith strength hope and wisdom.

I think God done for me what I could not do for my self.

I got a great sense of comfort in knowing and believing that god was, and still is my partner.

I genuinely asked for help and I genuinely believe I got it.

I tried to turn to my left side, and out of nowhere a sharp agonising pain ran from under my arm down as far as my toes. It felt like a bunch of nettles were stinging me all down my left side.

I roared in pain.

Instantly the pretty nurse appeared at the side of my bed, and asked me what the problem was.

I told her of my pain. She said, "No problem Tony I will sort out some pain killers out for you."

She walked over to her stainless steel medication trolley in the corner of the ward and quietly fumbled around for a short while.

She returned to me and handed me three tablets, two pain killers and a sleeping tablet.

I popped them in my mouth and washed them down with a glass of water and within ten minutes the pain had eased off.

By now I was feeling drowsy and struggling to keep my eyes open.

I removed my Rosary Beads from my neck and wrapped them around my wrist, and I held the cross tightly in my hand. I began to pray myself to sleep.

I drifted off to sleep with only heavenly thoughts on my mind.

Chapter Twelve:

Back on My Feet

I was woken by the words, "Wakie wakie."

My eyes were still closed as I assessed the level of pain I was feeling.

I scored myself at three out of ten. I was beginning to make a habit of this scoring system.

I was feeling good after a sound nights sleep.

As I opened my eyes, I realised my mind was not in a panicked state. I concluded that my life was not in immediate danger.

I felt strong enough to have a breakfast.

There were lots of doctor's nurses, and nurse's aids buzzing around the ward, they all seemed to be in a frantic panic.

Suddenly I heard the words, "He's gone."

Instantly I understood that the old man three beds down had just passed away to the other world. He was taken from the ward, and that was the last I saw of him. I prayed for his soul as he left the ward.

This event scared the breath out of my lungs.

I lay back thinking it could have easily being me, but for the grace of god and his blessed Mother and all the powers that be.

The only thing on my mind now was to get out of this living morgue, as soon as it was physically possible.

The drama was over and the ward fell into a deep eerie silence for at least ten minutes. I clutched my beads tight in my right hand and prayed for this poor mans soul to get to heaven.

I was very saddened by this event. It made me think how precious each day hour and minute is to us all.

Suddenly the silence was broken by the squeaky wheels of the breakfast trolleys.

An elderly looking lady offered me some breakfast.

I said no, I was so shocked by this man dying so close to me, my hunger disappeared.

The lady offered me tea or coffee. I settled for coffee and enjoyed every last drop.

A half hour later Mister Murphy walked into the ward and came straight to my bed.

First he looked at my left side drainage bag and to my surprise said, "Tony your bag is empty."

He looked at my charts and said, "Tony we are going to remove the tube and bag from your side." I was over the moon because every thing seemed to be going my way. I said please do.

He sat on the bed and said, "I am surprised that there is no blood in the bag." Yes I said a mini miracle.

He than looked at my pee bag and said, "I suppose you want that taken out as well."

O please I said. He told me the sister would arrange removal of the tubes shortly. He rose from the edge of my bed and said, "See you tomorrow," and proceeded on to the next patient.

I lay there and I was thrilled to bits but every second seemed like an hour.

Eventually a Pakistani doctor and two young and pretty Irish nurses were at my bedside.

One of the nurses handed me a tube of cream and told me to rub some on my wee little man. As they left the ward I pulled the sheet over my head for some privacy.

I rubbed the cream on and within ten minutes these three invaders were back at my bedside.

The doctor pulled the curtains around the bed, and the nurse pulled the sheet back. The doctor slowly pulled the tube from my little man, the pain was pure torture.

Eventually through sheer agony all the connections were removed.
This painful incident is etched on my memory for ever.
My three persecutors left as fast as they arrived.
Secretly I hoped I would never see them again.

I lay there thinking of God and our partnership.
I felt I had put up a good fight, a fight for my life and somehow I had obtained the first victory on my journey true and beyond can-sir.

I accepted I had confided in the heavens above and by doing so I obtained strength, courage, patience, and wisdom.
I put my trust in the mercy of Jesus and the Holy Spirit and they were merciful to me.
The health and strength of my soul was truly nourished by my daily prayers and meditation.
Suddenly my cell phone rang, I answered. It was Mary.
I was happy to hear her voice.

She waffled on for a while and then said, "Tony I am getting the three o clock train from Wexford, and I should be there by six o clock."
She asked me was there anything that I wanted.
I said just a few of my books. She said, "No problem Tony consider it done."
We said see ya later and we both hung up.

I called one of the nurses over to me and asked her could I get out of the bed for a small walk.
She told me she would have to check with the ward sister.
Ten minutes later the ward sister arrived at my bed, and said in a sarcastic manner, "What's this I hear about you wanting to go for a walk mister Power, do you think you are able."

Of course I am able sister I only lost my kidney not my legs or brain suddenly blurted out of my mouth.

Then she said, "I will talk to Mister Murphy and if he agrees with it, you can go ahead with your wee walk."

She vanished from the ward.

Twenty minutes or so passed by and out of the nurse's station came Mister Murphy.

As he approached he smiled at me and said out loud, "I suppose you want to do the River Dance next."

I grinned and said if you let me I will give it a go.

Mister Murphy sat on the side of my bed and asked me was I in pain, "Now answer me and tell the truth Tony."

Look I said I need to get some exercise and a breath of fresh air. He said, "That's not the answer I was looking for."

I than told him on a pain score it would probably be a five out of ten.

Right so he said, "Put your slippers on and off you go."

He left the ward.

I put my granddad cardigan on, and with a great struggle I leaned over the edge of my bed and slipped my slippers on my feet.

I rose to my feet and with great internal excitement; I took my first few steps.

Really it was more of a shuffle than a walk.

As I was shuffling my way to the entrance of the ward my eyes caught sight of an elderly man opposite me lying on his bed beside a big Georgian window.

We both made eye contact and smiled at each other, and not a word was spoken between us.

He raised his hand and stuck his thumb high in the air.

I appreciated his jester and shuffled on out of the ward.

I walked to the main door and walked outside.

As I took a deep breath of fresh air, I felt a sense of pure joy freedom and bliss.

I stared at the church across the road, and suddenly I felt a surge of excitement from deep within, all discomfort and torment temporarily left my body and mind.

A middle aged woman suddenly turned to me and said, "Would you like an apple."

I accepted it and thanked her.

As I was munching at the apple my eyes caught sight of too portly figures in the distance. Their shapes and their stride were familiar to me. I looked again, and this time I was sure it was my dad and my older brother. I saw them but I was sure they did not see me.

I slipped behind a large column, and I waited for them to arrive at the steps of the hospital.

As they walked up the steps, I calmly shuffled my body from behind the column, to greet them to my temporary home.

When they saw me they both nearly jumped out of their skin.

My dad hugged me and said, "Thank god you are ok Tony."

My brother asked me what I was doing outside.

I told him that I was disconnected from all the tubes about half an hour earlier and I needed some fresh air.

I finished my apple and we three slowly walked back to Saint Anthony's ward.

As I got back into bed a tremendous pain engulfed my newly fresh sown scar. I let out a roar and within a few seconds a small Pilipino nurse was at my bed side.

She asked my dad and brother to leave.

She told them to come back in fifteen minutes.

The nurse smiled at me and said, "Too far too soon."

She gave me a glass of water and two morphine tablets.

I popped them in my mouth and within ten minutes the pain began to ease off. Dad and my brother appeared about half an hour later.

They sat on either side of my bed and we chatted away for what seemed like an hour.

My dad asked me where the toilets were. I told him and off he went.

My brother than told me he had a few heavy words with dad on the train up. I asked him what it was about.

My brother said, "Tony it was all about the way we were reared up." Life was hard when we were young dad was fond of his alcohol and there were many a row between mum and him over it. My home back then was not a nice place to be for a child. The police were regulars at our door. I looked at my brother and

I said will you let it go for now. He replied, "I let it go on the train." "I asked him for an apology and Tony he sincerely apologised."

My dad returned and sat on the chair beside the bed.

He looked at me with tears in his eyes and said, "Tony I am so sorry for all the pain and trouble I caused the whole family through my drinking."

I told him that was in the past and it has no relevance in the here and now.

By now all this emotional stuff was disturbing the little bit of serenity that I had left in my soul.

I told them that I was very tired and that I needed to go to sleep.

They bid me farewell and left on their journey back to Waterford City.

I lay their motionless gathering my thoughts and regaining my mental composure, for at least ten minutes.

As I looked at my watch on the locker. I could hear the squeaky wheels of the dinner trolley being pushed along.

I was given a lovely meal of chicken mashed potatoes and peas.

I enjoyed every last pea on the plate. For afters I was given jelly and ice cream.

The jelly and ice cream was out of this world.

With a full belly and a weary body, I drifted off to sleep.

The sound of my phone ringing suddenly woke me.

I answered and I was thrilled to bits to hear the voice of Theresa my earthly Angel from America. She asked how I was feeling. I told her every thing went well, and I thanked her for all her work and time she had spent knee deep in scans and medical reports for me. She told me that they had lit some candles as my surgery was going on, and that they sent me pure white light. I thanked her from the bottom of my heart.

I said goodbye and God bless, and Theresa said, "Wait a minute Paul wants to speak to you."

A few seconds passed by and Paul said in a deep American voice, "Top of the morning to you Tony." I replied in a thick Irish accent and said, top of the morning to you to Paul.

Paul asked me was their anything that I needed. I said no you have done too much for me all ready. He replied. "Tony stay well and keep breathing, and if you need anything and I mean anything just ring Theresa." Paul said, "Tony As soon as you are well again get your ass back here, and it's my treat for a good Irish man.

I thanked him again for his generosity and said God bless and hung up.

By now I was feeling very tired so I cuddled into Kidney and drifted off to sleep.

Two hours later Mary woke me up with a gentle kiss on my face. I looked at my watch; it was seven in the evening.

Mary offered to get me a Star Bucks coffee I accepted and Mary disappeared from the ward.

Fifteen minutes later Mary returned with the coffee.

I called the nurse to my bed and asked her could I go out side for some fresh air. To my amazement she said, "Yes mister Power."

I moved myself to the side of my bed and Mary handed me my slippers.

I slipped them on and we walked slowly towards the main door of the hospital.

A short distance from the ward I noticed two patients coming up a side stairwell.

I stopped them and asked them where the smoking area was. Without words one of them just pointed to the bottom of the stairs.

Mary linked my arm as we made our way down the stairs and into the courtyard.

As we entered the yard I was amazed and amused to see, nurses, doctors, patients and visitors, so many people smoking in the one area.

We sat on a window ledge and sipped our coffee and smoked our cigarettes. They both tasted like a gift from above.

Suddenly a tall man in his early thirty's approached me and asked me for a light. I gave him my lighter and he lit an extra long cigarette. The second he lit it I could smell cannabis.

He gave me my lighter back and asked me did I want a smoke of his joint. I said yes as Mary stared at me in disbelief.

The tall man handed me the joint. I took a few pulls and almost instantly I was stoned off my face.

The man asked me what I was in hospital for. I told him kidney can-sir.

I asked him what he was here for. He told me that he had Aids.

I was instantly shocked annoyed and scared.

Now there was a possibility I would have to deal with Aids on top of can-sir.

Mary linked my arm and we walked around the court yard for at least ten minutes, and we finished our coffee. By now my head was starting to clear from the smoke.

We slowly made it back to Saint Anthony's ward.

I got straight into my bed and pulled the covers over my head, I felt semi paralysed.

I prayed to God to spare me from possible Aids.

Mary reached under the sheet and pinched my arm and said, "Tony for Gods sake cop on and get your head together."

I pulled the sheet back and looked at Mary and said you're right.

We intensely stared at each other for a brief few moments than we hugged each other.

Mary asked me what it was like here. I told her the staff are super and the food is even better.

We chatted about trivial things for an hour or so.

By now I was nodding in and out of sleep, and Mary was tired after her long trip to the Mater hospital.

Mary kissed me gently on the cheek and said, Good boy and God bless, and then she left the hospital.

As I lay their on my own I put my hand over my fresh wound and thanked the God of my understanding for my life. I also felt a sense of loss. I guess this feeling was due to the total loss of my left kidney. One good thing flashed across my mind, and that was I had the ability to pe pe at will.

Suddenly my mind drifted to the not so far away future, and to tell the truth I was scared big time of the surgery that I was booked in for in thirty days time.

I wondered how strong I could make myself before the next surgery.

As I thought about the next surgery goose pimples appeared on the back of my neck and arms, and the hair stood up on my head. I wondered would I survive it.

I saw this upcoming surgery as the greatest war of my life so far.

Suddenly my thoughts were interrupted by the squeaky wheels of the medication trolley doing its rounds of the wards.

I looked to my right side and I could see an attractive petite Irish nurse approaching my bed.

From a short distance away the attractive nurse said, "Hello Mister Power how are you doing."

I told her I was feeling tired and in a small bit of pain from my wound.

The nurse opened her trolley and fumbled around for a few seconds, and than she handed me two pain killers and a sleeping tablet.

I popped them in my mouth and clutched my Rosary Beads tightly in the palm of my hand, and I began to pray. I guess within ten to fifteen minutes it was lights out for me.

I was awakened at about six o clock in the morning by a loud metal crashing noise. I looked towards the floor near the end of the ward, and I could see a bed pan turned up side down and pe pe all over the floor. It was quickly dealt with by the pretty nurse and her aid.

The ward soon got back to normal. I snuggled into Kidney as I lay there trying to go back to sleep but my anxious mind was not having any of it.

I said the Rosary a few times and this seemed to squash my anxious mind.

Time passed quickly as I prayed.

All of a sudden it was breakfast time the breakfast trolleys were in top gear.

The nurse's aid offered me a small Irish breakfast and coffee or porridge and toast and tea.

I said I will have the lot please.

I could see that the nurse's aid was a little bit shocked but she gave me the two breakfasts any way.

I munched them down and I was feeling content and full.

Pretty soon after breakfast I was told by the pretty little nurse, that there would be a nurse's aid along to take me for a wash. I secretly hoped they would be a man.

Within ten minutes the aid arrived at my bed and introduced herself as Noreen, she asked me was I ready for a wash and blow dry and a scrub up.

I told Noreen I was a bit shy and embarrassed. She grinned at me and said, "Get in the wheel chair Mister Power," and in a joking manner she said, "If you don't hurry up all the hot water will be gone."

I got in the wheel chair and I was pushed to the wash room.

Noreen asked me to take my p.jays off, and I did but all the time I was covering my little man with my hand.

Noreen scrubbed me from head to toe, as if she was naturally washing one of her own children.

She dried me off and helped me get into my clean p.jays.

On the way back to the ward Noreen asked me did I smoke I didn't answer her. I just pointed to the main door.

She pushed my wheel chair and me in it, to the door.

I got up from my chair and walked out side.

Noreen passed me a lighted cigarette.

I took a few puffs and I felt a bit light headed, but that didn't stop me from finishing my smoke.

When our smoke was finished Noreen pointed at the wheel chair. I instantly knew what she meant and I obeyed her, and within five minutes I was comfortable sitting back in my bed.

Ten minutes later Mister Murphy and Mister Akiatar entered the ward on their daily rounds.

After half an hour or so, they were at my bed.

Mister Murphy plucked my charts from the end of the bed and briefly looked at it, and then he handed it to Mister Akiatar.

They both took a few steps back from my bed and started to talk in big words that I could not understand. The two surgeons stepped back to my bed side.

Out of nowhere Mister Murphy said, "Tony you're going home tomorrow and we will talk tomorrow before you go."

I was a bit shocked but I was instantly over the moon. The surgeons disappeared to the next bed.

Within a few minutes I lay back on the bed and began to pray and give thanks to the creator for helping me mentally, and physically through this first bad cancerous period.

I wondered to myself how strong I could get my body for the next surgery in thirty days time. I knew there and than that life for me would never be the same again.

As I tried to hold on to my mental composure I wondered is it a psychiatric hospital I should be going to instead of home.

Suddenly my mobile phone rang I answered, it was Mary.

She asked me how I was feeling. I told her I was over the moon and I was going home tomorrow. She did not believe me at first, she seemed bamboozled.

Ten minutes later and Mary arrived at the ward with Star Bucks coffee for me.

I got out of bed and Mary and I made our way down the stairs into the court yard. We sat on a window sill and sipped our coffee and smoked our cigarettes. We wandered around the hospital for at least half an hour, and then we returned to my hospital ward. I got back into bed and to tell the truth my body was all maxed out. Mary than asked me, how are we going to get home tomorrow.

I asked Mary to take the six o clock train home to Wexford; she agreed and said, "How in the name of god are you going to get home."

I told Mary that my younger sister and her husband were driving up to see me tomorrow, and I would hitch a lift back home from them. Mary stayed chatting with me for at least two hours, and than she said her good byes and left to catch the Wexford train. I was excited and giddy at the thoughts of going home within the next twenty four hours. Time passed slowly that evening, every minute felt like an hour. As I lay in my hospital bed my thoughts and feelings were running amuck. I found it very hard to focus and centre my thoughts.

I was trying to consider my future if I had any at all. I knew my future would be hard on me mentally and physically.

I also figured out that my own attitude and willingness to get well would play the biggest role in my recovery.

Just over a month ago I thought I would live to a ripe old age. Now I realise life must be lived only one day at a time.

Suddenly the phone in the nurse's station rang out. I could see the nurse picking it up through the glass windows of the station. She left the receiver on the desk and raced over to me, and told me that a Mister Fisher was on the phone. I slipped out of bed and walked to the phone. The first thing P.C. said to me was, "Turn you're flipping cell phone on Tony."

I apologised and told him it was hard to get a signal within the hospital walls. We chatted on for at least half an hour. I told P.C. that I was going home tomorrow, he paused in disbelief and after a few seconds said, "Tony you're a remarkable man keep your spirit above all your suffering and you will get well." We said farewell and God bless and hung up. I thanked the nurse and I walked back to my bed. I popped my slippers off and slid back into my bed. By now I was feeling very tired and worn out from the whole hospital experience. But I can honestly say this was the happiest evening I had spent in hospital so far.

I realised that night while deep in thought that I and my God had won our first major battle with Can- Sir, and it was more than what I had hoped and prayed for. Later on that night the nurse gave me my usual pain killers and a sleeping tablet. I asked for a second sleeping tablet and the kind nurse replied, "One should be good enough," she told me she could get into big trouble and even lose her job. As I lay there I guess I drifted off into a deep sleep.

Suddenly I woke up I looked at my watch on my locker it was six thirty A.M.

I tried to wander back to sleep but I was so excited and grateful to be going home. My mind was in overdrive.

The only way to calm my mind was to pray, and I closed my eyes and clutched my Rosary Beads and prayed in a positive manner.

After a half hour praying and giving thanks to the all mighty, I snapped out of my prayer like trance.

Suddenly it was breakfast time.

I was given a choice porridge and tea and toast or the big Irish fry. I opted for the fry and polished it off as if it was the last meal I would ever have.

I lay there in relative comfort. My newly made surgical wound was itchy.

I pulled the bed sheet over my head and reached down to scratch my wound.

I was shocked to see that the dressing had peeled away over night, only to reveal a long line of metal staples protruding from my fresh wound, starting at about an inch from my belly button, going nearly all the way around my back.

This sight scared the living day light out of me.

I quickly pulled the bed sheet down, and decided I needed a new dressing on my wound.

I called the nurse over to my bed and showed her my ruffled up dressing. The nurse looked at my scar and to my amazement said, "Tony that's the fastest I have ever seen a wound healing."

Those words that morning gave me hope and strength to carry on my journey through and beyond can-sir.

When I entered the Mater hospital I was full of fear and despair, now this kind nurse with just a few sweet kind words had infused me with a bit of hope and confidence in myself, and in my healing ability from within.

The kind nurse that morning sparked something special within me.

The nurse than said, "Tony there is no point in putting a new dressing on because the doctors will be here within a half hour." I said thanks a million as she left my bed side.

As I lay their waiting for the doctors my thoughts deepened. I realised I must have one powerful guardian Angel looking over and after me.

Time passed by slowly every minute felt like an hour to me.

Eventually after what seemed like a life time Mister Murphy and Mister Akiatar entered the ward, and came straight over to me.

Mister Murphy said, "How is the man from the Crystal City?"

I replied I think I am ready willing and able to go home now.

Mister Murphy pulled my bed covers down, and stared at my wound for a minute or so in silence.

The first words out of his mouth were, "Tony you have great healing powers you're a very lucky man."

I replied thank God and his Blessed Mother.

Mister Murphy than told me they needed blood tests and he said, "If all is well you're on your way home today."

I told him my sister and her husband were on their way up to visit me, and I could travel home with them. He replied, "Tony it all depends on your blood results."

The two surgeons looked at me and they both had big smiles on their faces. I really didn't know why they were smiling at me, but I presume they were happy with their successful surgery on me.

Mister Murphy beckoned the nurse over and asked her to do bloods on me, than the two surgeons moved on to the next patient.

I lay my head down and willed the bloods to be on the money, and then I snuggled into kidney for some quite time and comfort.

By this time I was infused with a small glimmer of hope, and now I understood deep inside my heart and soul, that some hope is better than no hope at all.

Somehow it felt like I got a reprieve from my executioner.

My stay in hospital had caused me pain with twisted thoughts. There was a time their when I doubted my own strengths and courage, thank God and his Blessed Mother that this time had passed by.

As I lay their staring at the dark pattern ceiling a Pilipino nurse entered the ward with her bloods trolley, and came straight to my bed and smiled at me.

She said, "Show me your arm." I did and suddenly with accuracy and a steady hand she plunged the needle into my right arm and drew blood.

She filed three small vials and capped them off.

Honestly I felt like a vampire had punctured my skin and drew blood. She told me that the results would be back in about an hour, and then she left the ward.

I put my head down on the pillow and tried to relax but it was near impossible. All sorts of negative rubbish entered my head.

I wondered how long I had left to live.

I fumbled around my bed and eventually I found my Rosary Beads hanging off the side of the bed.

I grabbed them and began to pray from deep within my heart soul and mind.

As I prayed I asked God to help me identify what areas in my life needed changing in order to get well and stay well.

I asked God in earnest was it possible to re-program me.

Suddenly I rose from my bed and knelt down and said the Our Father, and than I popped myself back into the bed.

I continued praying until suddenly Mister Murphy appeared at my bedside again with charts under his arm.

I looked at him face to face and he smiled at me and said, "Tony I am pleased to tell you that your bloods are fine you can pack your bags you are going home." I think my heart stopped for a second with pure excitement and joy.

Mister Murphy than asked me had I any questions. I said yes, and I asked him what medication I would be on.

He laughed at me and said, "No meds just water and lots of it at least three litres a day Tony, for the rest of your life."

I thanked him and we shook hands and then he said, "Be back here in a month's time and we will go to plan B."

I had no need or want to know what plan B was at that moment.

Mister Murphy then left the ward.

Straight away I switched the cell phone on and rang my sister, and I asked her was she still coming up to visit me. She told me that they were about an hour away. She could sense I was excited and asked me was I alright.

I told her I was fine and that she had an extra passenger for the journey back home.

She asked me was I serious! I replied one hundred and ten percent serious. I asked my sister would she collect me at the main entrance of the hospital when she arrived. "No bother" she said and we hung up.

I packed the bits and pieces that I had gathered in hospital. I jumped out of my P.Jays and put my new clothes on. I said my goodbyes and left the ward and walked towards the main door of the hospital.

I could smell coffee and I got a compulsion to get one.

I purchased the coffee and quickly made my exit.

I sat on my bag and lit a cigarette and sipped my coffee.

I was over the moon to be alive and still living in this mad and crazy world.

I lit a second cigarette and closed my eyes, and I thanked the powers that be for my strength and courage through this first part of my journey.

When I opened my eyes my sister and her husband were standing right in front of me. I was thrilled to bits to see them there so soon.

Chapter Thirteen:
A Journey Within Itself

I hugged my younger sister as she shed some tears. I asked her what's wrong she replied, "Tony they are tears of joy I am happy you're alive."

My sisters husband Tom said, "Let's get on the road I don't want to get stuck in heavy traffic."

We walked to the car park and Tom put my stuff in the boot and got in the car.

Before we drove off my sister passed me a bundle of envelopes.

I asked her what's this all about. She replied, "Tony they are Mass cards and get well soon cards from neighbours and friends in Waterford." Tom drove out of the car park and as he did I started to open the envelopes.

Each one I read and I placed it on the seat beside me. I hadn't finished opening them all and all of a sudden I got very weepy and grateful all at the same time. I tried to steady my thoughts and hold back the tears but that day it was impossible to do so.

Somehow for a few moments I sensed and felt the power of other peoples prayers and get well wishes.

It encouraged me deep inside to be positive and optimistic for the future.

Now I know that all prayers work on a level that we as human beings don't fully understand.

I opened the next envelope and to my surprise the card on the inside read enjoy and the outside read get well soon there were no names on it.

There was also a small parcel in the envelope.

I opened the parcel and to my amazement it was a small bag of weed.

I told my sister and her husband of my find. They both laughed out loud.

Tom then turned his head towards me and said, "Tony make one up for yourself, and as soon as we get out of Dublin I will stop and you can enjoy the rest of the journey home."

Suddenly my cell phone rang I answered it, and it was Mary. She asked was I still in the hospital. I told her I was in the car and on the way down home.

I told her that I missed her big time and I can't wait to hug and kiss her, she said the same.

I told Mary we would arrive at about six o clock.

Mary asked me what I would like for dinner.

I answered her and said a big Irish sloppy stew would be wonderful. She said, "Consider it done Tony" and we hung up.

Twenty minutes passed by and we were now on the outskirts of Dublin. Tom pulled the car into a lay by and said, "Tony fire up your joint."

I got out of the car and lit the joint and took four or five pulls of it and then put it out.

I got back in the car and my head started to spin but I felt no pain and I felt very happy and warm on the inside.

My sister and Tom looked at me and burst out laughing.

I asked what's up lads as their laughing increased.

Tom said, "Tony your face is pure red and your eyes are like the red on the traffic lights."

Tom started the car and we drove on.

After a short while I lay back on the back seat of the car and drifted off into a deep narcotic sleep.

Suddenly I was wakened by a dog barking I opened my eyes and Lana was on her two back legs scratching at the window of the car.

I got out of the car and with great effort I lay down on the ground and cuddled into Lana.

Mary and her three children heard all the commotion, and quickly made their way to the front gates.

We had a big group hug, and then we all went into Mary's house.

As I entered I could smell a wonderful smell of cooking.

We all sat down at the kitchen table and chatted for a while.

As we were chatting Mary dressed the table, and five minutes later Mary dished up the best Irish stew that I ever had in my life. Twenty minutes later my sister and her husband left for Waterford.

I hadn't heard from my son Shane in a few days, this made me uneasy and unsettled within myself. I left the kitchen and went out to the Grotto at the end of Mary's garden. I rang Shane and told him I was doing fine and I am still breathing.

I could tell by his loud voice that he was over the moon to be talking to me.

I told Shane to give me a few days to get well and I would be down to spend some time with him. Shane said, "Dad take as long as it takes to get well."

We said good bye and God bless to each other and hung up.

I knelt down that mid October frosty night and lit three candles, and I began to thank the God of my understanding for his Mercy towards me.

I pulled my Beads from my pocket and proceeded to pray the Rosary. After a few moments passed by, uncountable tears burst from my eyes like never before, this was the first good cry I had on my own since my surgery.

They were not tears of grief or sadness; they were tears of pure joy and happiness and contentment, and a small bit of bliss.

Right there and then I understood that I had some mega force guiding me in the right direction. I wondered where all this power was coming from.

As I was praying Lana suddenly appeared at my side. I sat on the bench at the grotto, and Lana popped her self up beside me.

I snuggled into Lana, and I left my mind wander on to Godley things.

I briefly looked back through the last week in my mind and I suddenly realised I had BEEN TO HELL and the key word here was BACK AGAIN.

At that moment I felt like a light of hope was surrounding me, and protecting my sanity through this jungle of can-sir.

That cold and frosty October night in 2004 while at the grotto, I felt like I was on the way to rekindling my damaged spirit.

I thanked the creator and the universe for giving me a temporary escape route from a horrible death.

I opened my eyes to the truth of can-sir and accepted it, and as soon as I did a lot of my fears vanished from within my mind that night.

I was starting to shiver from the cold so Lana and I returned to the house. I opened the back door and the blast of heat was beautiful.

I went into the house and I told Mary's children some good ghost stories for at least an hour, and then Mary sent them off to bed.

We went to the sitting room to watch some television.

Well I was in hospital Mary had rearranged the sitting room. She put a small camp bed in the corner of the room so I could lie there and watch the television and get well.

By now after such a long and drawn out day the pain started creeping back into to my wound.

I took two pain killers and lay down on the camp bed, and the pain eased off within ten minutes.

Lana jumped up on the bed and wiggled herself into the comfort zone, and within a few minutes that was it. I fell into a deep sleep that lasted till seven the next morning.

I tried to get out of bed but any sudden movement caused me intense pain in the surgery site.

I lay back down and I tried to compose myself.

I lay dead still and I began to pray.

I can remember my first prayer that day, and it went like this.

Thank you God for this day,

Please help this pain go away.

As I continued praying I felt like I was tucked under the wings of the universe.

I thanked God for the ability to deal with my reality and my reality was can-sir.

I thought to myself at least my faith was the strongest weapon that I had, and I felt my Faith was in my hands, heart, soul and mind.

I realised now that miracles do happen, and I told myself there was no way I was going to face a lingering death.

I know that the chips were down, and every moment was precious to me, but that morning I understood that the strongest emotion within me was self preservation.

I was not yet ready, and I did not wish to travel on the road to eternity yet.

I know now that one of my problems was, I was looking out to much and really I should have being looking within.

I know now that I wanted a peaceful and loving existence. I know that self love is the most important love, and I feel this love has the power to go inside and affect changes.

This love for me was like a stepping stone on the road to getting well again.

By now Mary and her children were scurrying around the house preparing for school. As soon as I heard them I forced myself beyond my pain and got of my camp bed. I unsteadily walked to the kitchen.

As soon as I walked in the children greeted me and Mary hugged and kissed me.

Mary whispered with a stern voice, "Tony what in the name of God are you doing, get back to your bed right now."

I said one word to Mary and that was coffee, and I left the kitchen as fast as I entered.

I jumped back into the camp bed and within five minutes Mary came in with Star Bucks coffee that she had purchased while in Dublin.

I was thrilled to bits but the only thing missing was a cigarette. I told Mary I needed a smoke and for the first time since diagnosis Mary said, "Do you think that's wise."

I replied I don't care at this very moment.

Mary opened the window and said, "Fire away to your hearts content."

With great difficulty I eased myself towards the window and lit my cigarette and sipped my star buck's coffee, hand in hand they were glories.

Mary noticed that I was in pain, and she asked me did I take my pain killers. I said not yet. She told me that the sooner I take them the sooner the pain will disappear.

Mary than told me she was leaving for the school, and after dropping the children of that she was heading for Wexford town to do food shopping. Five minutes later they all said good bye and left the house.

I got my pain killers and popped two into me, and twenty minutes later I felt a small bit better and fully awake.

With great difficulty and a massive physical effort I took a shower, and afterwards I felt clean and ready for the day ahead.

I tried ringing my son Shane but I got no answer. I guess he was still in bed.

I made some toast and tea for myself, and I gave Lana a can of dog food and a bowl of water.

When Lana finished eating I decided to walk to the grotto at the end of the garden, Lana walked by my left side to the grotto.

I suddenly sensed that Lana sensed the sight of my surgery. I tried to walk her on my right side but she kept re positioning herself on my left side.

I sat on the rocks beside the Grotto, and Lana lay on the grass beside me.

I said a decade of the rosary and then slowly and painstakingly walked back to the house.

That day I felt privileged to just be able to walk.

My short excursions had partly worn me out so I decided to go back to bed. I switched the T.V. on, and Lana and I popped back up on the camp bed.

I tried to make Lana lie by my good side but she kept drifting back to my surgery site.

I drifted off to sleep and I presume Lana did as well.

Suddenly I was disturbed by car doors banging and loud children.

I looked out the window, Mary and her children had arrived home. I got out of bed and opened the front door for them.

Mary said in an agitated voice, "Tony what in the name of god are you doing out of bed."

I told her that I was in bed for most of the day sleeping.

Mary advised me to get back into bed, so I did exactly what I was told.

The pain was creeping back in my side so I popped two pain killers and lay back down.

After about twenty minutes passed I called Mary and asked her to leave the children in to me.

She agreed and said, "Tony only for a half hour."

The children and Lana came in, and the mood of the room changed from quietness to pandemonium.

Mary left out a roar from the kitchen and told us all to quieten down.

I asked the children to quieten down, and to give them their due they suddenly did.

Suddenly in the quietness of the room Mary's youngest child Adam who was six at the time jumped up on the camp bed and put his face close to my ear and said, "Tony I have two kidneys you can have one of mine."

I was dumb struck but somehow infused with hope for the future, to hear such a genuine offer from a young kid. With great effort I held back my tears.

Adam then asked me could I show him the big owee.

I told him that I would have to ask his mother first.

He jumped of the bed and went to Mary in the kitchen, and I presume he asked her the same question.

He returned and said, "Mammy said yes."

He propped himself up along side me in the bed and said, "Show me the owee."

I slowly removed the dressing to reveal the long line of staples.

Adam stared at my wound and said, "Holy God make it better Tony." His words were so sincere and powerful, and meaningful and uplifting to me.

I could sense the raw simplicity of this child's faith and belief.

Adams words were so valuable to me.

I asked the children to leave the room, because I needed to absorb what was just said to me. I told the children I needed some rest and they unwillingly left the room.

Five minutes passed by and Mary called me for dinner.

With a bit of effort I made my way to the kitchen and sat down as fast as I could, for I was feeling weak and weary.

Mary dished up steak and chips and peas it was delicious and full of protein, just what I needed to pick my energy levels up.

It was truly the nicest meal I had since Boulder City Nevada.

As I rose from the table I felt a tremendous pain in my tummy, and I instantly sat down and put my hands on my belly. I tried to keep a happy face on but it was near impossible.

Mary looked at me and pointed towards the sitting room. I rose from the chair and slowly made my way to the camp bed and lay down, and as I did I realised I had eaten too much food.

The pain felt like my tummy was touching the inside of my wound.

Mary came in and asked me was I all right.

By now drops of sweat were pouring from my face.

Mary said, "Tony it looks like your constipated."

I asked Mary had she any thing in the house to sort out this problem.

Mary did not answer me. She left the room and within a minute she returned with a bottle of extra virgin olive oil.

She handed it to me and said, "Tony drink as much as you can, this will clear your system out within ten minutes."

I slugged a big gulp of it and within five minutes I was heading to the loo. All as I can say to my self about that episode was thank God and his Blessed Mother the bomb had dropped.

I returned to the camp bed feeling relieved and at ease within my belly.

About seventy percent of the pain was gone, and this allowed me to relax and watch television in relative comfort for the rest of the evening

Mary was preparing the children for bed and I lay back on my camp bed.

The three children came into me. I hugged them and said good night and god bless.

Mary hauled them out of the sitting room and put them to bed.

Ten minutes passed and the whole house fell into a peaceful silence.

Suddenly the door opened and Mary entered the sitting room with two cups of coffee she passed me one, and sat beside me on the camp bed.

Mary asked me how I was coping in my head.

That night I told Mary that I was scared of the upcoming surgery. I also told Mary that I did not think I had enough time to recuperate before the next big operation.

Mary said, "Tony it seems like you are feeling sorry for yourself, please take it day by day, and you'll be fine."

Mary told me a lovely uplifting little story and it went like this,

I felt sorry for myself because I had no shoes, until I met a man who had no feet.

These few words made me realise that I am still alive, and I must appreciate things a lot more in the here and now.

I realise I had great doubts and fears about the upcoming surgery. I wondered would I be dead in a month's time or less.

Can-sir had produced a lot of unbearable and unrelenting thoughts in my mind.

Mary kissed me and said, "God Bless," and left the room to go to bed.

As soon as she left the room my mind wandered back into negativity.

I wondered what almighty force would be guiding me from this place to the next.

I thought of an escape route out of this living hell, and I briefly contemplated suicide but not seriously thank God.

That night I felt like a piece of dying meat.

I thought to myself, another day coming to an end, and Tony is another day deeper in "DEATH."

I realised that night that my original positive outlook was fading only to reveal nasty stinking thinking.

I got out of bed knelt down and began to pray.

I remember clearly saying,

O holy one in Heaven and in me please help me find who I am, and who I want to be, and who you want me to be.

I got back into bed and from my brief chat with the holy one, the mental strain on my brain had eased slightly.

I don't drink alcohol but that night I felt I could prop up the bar somewhere all on my own.

Suddenly I realised I still had some cannabis.

I made myself a joint, and silently made my way to the front porch.

I lit the joint and within five minutes my mind had switched to different thought patterns.

I sat down on a small bench outside the front door, and in that moment I felt truly happy no matter what the future would bring.

It seemed like the cannabis vanished my fears and thoughts and anxieties from my mind, if only temporary.

Suddenly I could hear Lana scratching at the door.

I opened the door and Lana bullied her way out.

I grabbed her collar and guided us to the Grotto.

I sat with Lana and I prayed the Rosary twice that night.

Lana and I returned to the house, and I went for a pe pe.

I quietly made my way to the camp bed and lay down and began to pray myself to sleep.

In what seemed like an instant I was awake again.

I looked at my watch and to my amazement it was seven o clock in the morning.

Strange as it may seem I felt fresh as a daisy and ready for the day ahead.

I quickly rose from my bed and took Lana for a pe pe.

I went back in to the house and the children were up and running about getting ready for school.

We all sat down and had some cereal for our breakfast.

Mary asked me what plans I had for the day.

I told her I just wanted to chill out and do some reading and praying for the day.

Mary replied, "Tony that sounds like a good idea."

I asked Mary what she was going to do and she said "Shopping." Then she asked me would I like to come with her I said no I need to relax and get my strength back.

Mary and the children put their coats scarves and gloves on, and said bye bye and left for school and shopping. An eerie silence fell over the house.

By now the pain in my scar was increasing by the minute. I decided to take two pain killers, ten minutes later and the pain started to dissipate.

I called out to Lana and in seconds she was by my side. I grabbed her lead from behind the door and we walked out onto the old country road, and headed for the old train tracks. The walking was tiring painful and slow, but I persevered and we got there.

I sat down on the damp dewy grass by the railway gates, and I tried to gather my thoughts and feelings.

One of my deepest feelings was, I felt like I was a burden on Mary and her children, and I felt as time would pass by I would be a bigger burden on them.

This was something I did not want to put on anybody's shoulders.

I released Lana's lead and with great effort I climbed over the railway gate, and Lana crawled under.

We both wandered down the old railway line.

I stayed on the tracks, and Lana wandered in and out of the bushes on either side of the track. A mile or so down the track Lana disappeared. I called her name out lots of times, but she was nowhere to be found.

I wondered did she head home through the fields.

I kept walking on in the hope that I would find her, and then suddenly out of the corner of my left eye I could see her sitting in the bushes.

I called her but she would not come to me.

I sensed that she wanted me to go to her.

With a lot of effort, I made my way down the small embankment. I spread apart the bushes and I was overwhelmed and amazed by what was there.

Here was Lana sitting in a hidden and abandoned grotto along side an old weather beaten statue of Saint Patrick.

I knew instantly this was some sort of sign but I didn't know what it meant, but I knew it was a good sign.

I sat on a stone in this new found grotto and I thanked the universe for leading me here.

I prayed for a short while, and suddenly a sheer sense of peace and harmony covered my whole being.

I felt comfortable and at ease within myself.

Some how I felt that the powers that be, led me to this grotto of tranquillity, for healing and happiness within my distorted mind.

All the time I was there, I noticed Lana was staying dead still. I wondered to myself was she praying too, or did she feel some kind of presence at the Grotto of Saint Patrick, after all she was the one that found it.

Lana and I stayed there for at least an half an hour.

Eventually we embarked on our journey towards the house. It was slow slogging but I got there without too much pain.

As soon as I entered the house Lana went to the press where her food was kept. I gave Lana an extra helping, and as quick as I gave it to her she wolfed it down.

The morning had taken its toll on me and I needed to lie down.

I made a coffee and went to my camp bed and put my feet up.

I enjoyed my coffee and when I was finished I lay down and went into a deep sleep.

Suddenly my cell phone rang I answered it. I was delighted it was Shane my son.

I asked Shane was he o.k., he did not answer my question, but he said, "Are you all right dad."

All as I said to Shane was that everything was on the ball.

I told Shane that I would see him tomorrow before my appointment with Doctor Rowe in the morning, and after it again.

I said Shane thanks for being my son I love you to bits, and we will have a ball of a time tomorrow.

"I love you too dad see you then," and he hung up.

The rest of that day was pretty eventless, and by the end of it I was feeling bored and out of sorts with my brain.

Mary and the children returned to the house at roughly about five in the evening.

The children helped her bring the shopping in to the house. Mary put the dinner on, and within a half hour we were all well fed and full up.

The children and I loudly played around the house for a couple of hours, until Mary left out a scream and told us all to quieten down.

She also told the children to get ready for bed.

They obeyed her orders straight away.

Mary put the children to bed and the house became very quiet and peaceful. We sat down in the sitting room and I told Mary about the Grotto of Saint Patrick.

She seemed very surprised. Mary said, "Tony I suppose this is the same as the church, and the old woman in Dublin."

I told Mary I would bring her there tomorrow.

Mary suddenly got up and left the room and returned within two minutes with a small paper bag in her hand.

Mary passed the bag to me and I opened it and pulled the contents out.

To my surprise it was a bottle of ESSIAC and a packet of dried herbs.

Mary then told me to take it three times a day for the rest of your life.

I opened the bottle and swigged some down.

It tasted rank and mouldy but I understood that this was the American Indians way of curing can-sir.

Later on that night Mary and I decided to boil the ESSIAC herbs, and bottle the mixture for later use.

It was real fun and exciting boiling up, and making up your very own can-sir remedy. We went to bed and let the mixture soak over night. First thing the next morning we put the mixture into sterilised jam jars before the children were up out of bed.

Suddenly the children were up and running around getting ready for school and having their breakfast.

I took a shower and got dressed and told Mary I was heading for Waterford to see Doctor Rowe.

Mary said, "Are you driving."

I said yes.

Mary replied, "Tony you're off your head, are you out of your mind."

I told Mary that the driving would be no problem.

I said good bye and God bless and got into my car and drove off.

An hour and a half later I was in the waiting room in the doctor's clinic in Waterford. I waited twenty minutes and than I was called in.

Doctor Rowe greeted me and shook my hand, and said, "Pop up on the bed." I did and he slowly removed my dressing. He asked me when the staples were to be removed. I told him I did not know.

Suddenly he picked the phone up and requested the secretary to ring the Mater Hospital.

Five minutes later there was a knock on the door the secretary entered, and told the doctor that my staples were to come out today.

I was a bit surprised, and I was not mentally ready for this procedure.

Doctor Rowe rose from his chair and said, "Come with me Tony."

We walked to Doctor Creavin, s office, who is Doctor Rowe's partner in the practise. We entered her office and straight away she said, "Tony nice to meet you, I heard all about your journey from Mark."

I shook her hand and then she guided me to a small bed in the corner.

Doctor Rowe said, "Tony when your finished here call in to see me." I replied okey do and then he left the office.

I removed my coat and sat on the bed. I pulled my jumper up to my chest and I lay down on the bed.

with a gentle movement of her hands she stripped away the dressing. I did not feel a thing.

Doctor Craven then opened a small sealed bag of instruments; she held my hand and said, "Don't be so scared."

I lay their motionless, and with gentleness and a steady hand, she popped the first staple out.

Then she said, "Tony only sixteen more to go how are you feeling now."

I said I feel ok.

She carried on removing my staples and within a few minutes she had them all removed.

She asked me again how I was feeling.

I told her I was in a bit of pain but it was bearable.

To my surprise she told me that the wound was healing extremely fast.

She than dressed the wound and told me to keep it dry, and advised me to have a salt bath every day. I thanked her from the bottom of my heart.

As I was leaving her office she handed me a bundle of dressings and said, "Take care of your self Tony."

I said God Bless and I made my way to Doctor Rowe's waiting room. I sat down and within five minutes I was called in.

Doctor Rowe said Tony up on the bed.

I obeyed him straight away.

He gently pulled my jumper up and slowly peeled the mega plaster and stared at the scar for a brief moment.

He said, "Tony that looks brilliant." He really boosted my confidence in my self healing powers that day in his office.

He asked me how much pain I was in.

I told him the pain was a five out of ten.

He said that's not good.

He prescribed some pain killers and then said, "Tony come and see me any time you like, you don't need an appointment, just tell the girls at reception that you want to see Mark, they will have you flagged and you don't have to wait."

He also told me to stay away from old people and young children, and sick people.

In my naivety I asked him why.

He answered me and said, "Tony the can-sir and your surgery have weakened your immune system, and you are at a high risk of picking up germs of other people."

I told him about the book I was reading on herbs that heal, and that I came across herbs called Echinacea that is supposedly to increase the immune systems ability to deal with sickness.

Doctor Rowe looked at me and said, "Tony anything that you think works use it."

I thanked him from the bottom of my heart and left the practice.

I slowly made my way to the car park and got in to my car.

I turned the engine on, and the heater on full blast. I sat there on my own for at least ten minutes.

As I sat there I prayed and thanked the heavens for this day. Suddenly I realised that too much praying about the next life would not help me in this one. After all what's forty years compared to eternity.

The psychological challenge of trying to stay alive and live with can-sir was, and still is very tough on the brain.

I under stood that day, that the journey through and beyond can-sir, also can be a voyage of self discovery and enlightenment.

As I drove off to collect Shane I was feeling slightly more positive about my future.

I collected Shane, and with great difficulty and pain I drove to my home.

Shane helped me out of the car and shouldered me into the house.

I lay down on the couch and Shane tried to light a big fire for me. He made three efforts and eventually he had a roaring fire blasting out the heat. It was funny looking at him huffing and puffing as he tried to light the fire. Within ten minutes the sitting room was warm comfortable and cosy.

I tried to get up and the pain made it near impossible, and for some strange reason I was stuck to the couch.

Shane made me a coffee and gave me a few ginger nut biscuits. I was thrilled to bits by Shane's caring and kindness towards me.

I phoned Mary and told her of my mornings events.

I also told her that I was not able to drive because of the pain.

Mary said, "Tony you stay where you are and don't even attempt to drive the car until you are strong enough to do so."

As the day progressed I took two more painkillers, and they literally knocked me out and put me to sleep.

Suddenly I was awakened by the Angelus on the TV.

Before I fully opened my eyes I assessed my pain.

The pain killers had semi done their job. I sat up and Shane was sitting by the fire watching the television. I asked Shane was he hungry he said, "Yes dad."

I gave him some money and asked him to get me a fish and chip, and I told him to get what ever he wanted for himself.

Shane left the house and returned fifteen minutes later with the food.

We munched our food down and decided to watch a d.v.d.

Shane popped the MATRIX film in the d.v.d. player and we started to watch it.

Ten minutes later my pain was starting to increase so I took another two painkillers. I suppose they knocked me out cold. When I woke I was still on the couch, and it was five in the morning, it was very cold.

I got up and went straight to Shane's bed room. I looked in and I could see him all snuggled up in his bed, this sight made me feel wholesome for some weird reason. I went to my bedroom and I knelt down and said some prayers.

I got into bed and clutched my Rosary beads tightly in my right hand and I began to pray and meditate.

In my meditation I was projecting to a healthy and happy future.

I could see myself standing on a concrete sloped driveway, and I was wearing a white tee shirt and combat shorts, and white runners. I held this image in my mind as I drifted off to sleep again.

Suddenly my sleep was interrupted by Shane clattering around the house.

Before I got out of bed, I looked at my watch and to my amazement it was eleven o clock in the morning.

I called Shane and asked him what he was doing.

Shane replied, "Dad I am making you a big Irish breakfast."

I left Shane in the kitchen, and I went straight to the sitting room and plopped down on the couch.

Ten minutes later Shane gave me my big Irish breakfast.

I was truly overwhelmed because this was the first time that Shane had cooked for me.

I finished my breakfast and I was feeling a bit sore and agitated.

Shane rang his mum for a lift home.

Ten minutes later she was outside the house blowing the horn.

Shane said, "See you dad," and left the house.

I returned to the couch and propped myself up on some cushions.

I phoned Mary and told her it would take a week or so to get my strength back, if it comes back at all.

Mary said, "Tony stop being negative and start healing your self."

We spoke for at least ten minutes, and the last thing Mary said was, "Tony I hope you're taking the ESSIAC three times a day." I said yes but I was lying, I totally and genuinely forgot. We finished speaking and we hung up

I got up from the couch and with a big painful effort I lit a big coal fire. I tried to settle down and relax but my mind was starting to go into overdrive.

I was very worried and a bit scared about the next surgery, which was scheduled in less than three weeks time.

I seriously wondered were these my last three weeks on Earth.

It felt like my hope was slipping into the shadows of death.

For the next four days I stayed in my house and had the fire roaring constantly.

I started to read some of the books that Mary bought me in America, and I also dabbled into the Holy Bible which seemed to comfort and console my soul.

From my reading it felt like my self-belief and confidence and will power were being increased, the more I read the better I was feeling.

The days passed by and I had spent some quality time with my son.

The time passed quickly and I found myself on the road again heading for Wexford.

I arrived at Mary's house at about six thirty. It was a cold and dark night there was no moon in the sky.

I neglected to tell Mary that I was on my way down.

I stopped the car at the gates and got out. Suddenly Lana out of nowhere jumped all over me and licked the face off me.

I had to push her away.

Mary and the kids appeared at the front door and they were all excited to see me.

My timing was perfect Mary was dishing up the dinner.

I munched down the spaghetti Bolognese, and then I decided to go to the Grotto at the back of the garden.

I knelt down and I began to pray.

I asked the heavens above for the strength and wisdom to carry me through this horrible and sad period in my life.

When I finished praying I returned to the house.

By now the children were in bed and Mary was watching the television.

I told Mary that I was totally wiped out and I needed to lie down.

Mary pointed to the camp bed in the corner. I laid myself down and within five minutes I was out for the count.

The following morning I was lying in the camp bed wide awake and ready for the day. It was seven in the morning and Lana entered the sitting room. She jumped up on the camp bed. I snuggled into her for a few minutes.

I got out of bed and grabbed my coat and Lana's lead, and we walked out the front door.

It was a misty dark and damp morning and the sun was slow to make an appearance.

Lana and I walked the country road to the grotto of Saint Patrick by the old railway line.

I sat down and held my face in my hands, and I began to cry. I cried so much that morning it felt like a river had burst its banks wet tear drops were streaming from my face.

Suddenly the sun broke through the morning mist and for some strange reason, at that moment I felt re connected to the world. I had a strange feeling that morning; it felt like my body was wrapped in a shroud of mercy.

We left the grotto and walked off the railway tracks.

By now the sun was fully in view.

As I was walking I looked in the fields and saw some sheep grazing, and horses playing around, and for some strange reason I felt very close to God and nature.

As I walked on my thoughts deepened.

I thanked the God of my understanding for pulling me back from the border line of insanity and death.

I understood that morning that in the process of surviving the lows in life it bonded me closer to God.

That morning it felt like peace was flowing into my mind body soul and heart.

I understood that in God we can find support and courage to overcome our pain and suffering.

As I walked on I realised that the natural state in which body mind and soul work harmoniously, is a continuous replacement of energy that can only come from God.

Now I realise that joy and happiness and bliss, can spring from agony fear and despair.

I understood that I must keep in tune with the infinite power source from above, in order to get well again.

I realise that my soul will be at its peak when it adheres to God and his will for me.

As I walked towards the house I began to pray, and the first prayer in my mind was the serenity prayer which I feel I have to write down.

GOD GRANT ME THE SERINITY TO ACCEPT THE THINGS THAT I CAN NOT CHANGE THE COURAGE TO CHANGE THE THINGS THAT I CAN AND THE WISDOM TO KNOW THE DIFFERENCE. AMEN.

I continued praying as I walked the short distance to Mary's house.

As I arrived there Mary and the three children were getting in the car to go to school. I wished them well and than Mary said, "Tony I will be back in a half an hour."

They drove off and Lana and I went into the house.

I walked into the kitchen and the first thing I noticed, the table was empty except for one bottle of ESSIAC.

This was Mary's effort to make sure I took my herbs.

I opened the bottle and took a big slug. It tasted vile and earthy. I put the bottle in the fridge, and then went to my camp bed and lay down and tried to quieten my mind.

I snuggled into Kidney as I drifted off to sleep again.

Lana's sudden barking woke me up.

Mary had arrived back from the school.

We had a small breakfast together, and Mary was heading out again to the hair dressers.

I kissed her and said see you later. She went to her car and drove off.

I went to my camp bed and lay down, I clutched my beads again and I began to pray.

Suddenly I was disturbed by an alarm in the house next door. I got out of my bed and looked out the window. I could see through the neighbour's window, and I was shocked with the sight of flames of fire shooting up from the cooker wall. I hobbled my way to the front door and thumped on it for a couple of seconds, but no one answered.

I phoned the emergency services and told the operator what was going on.

She told me that the fire services were on their way, and because of the location of the house in the country it would take at least twenty minutes for them to get there.

I hung up the phone and I made my way to the back door.

I twisted the handle down and to my amazement the door opened.

I shouted as loud as I could. I bypassed the fire and made a quick search of the house.

The house was empty.

The flames from the cooker were shooting up the wall.

I went straight to the kitchen sink and grabbed some tea towels.

I quickly drenched them with water and placed them over the flames, they slightly quenched the flames.

I went back to the sink and grabbed the biggest pot that I could find. I filled it with water and I stood back a few feet from the cooker, and fired the water at the flames.

It took four more pots of water to extinguish the fire.

I looked at the cooker and the grill was glowing with heat.

I went to the fuse board in the hall and switched the power off. I went back to the kitchen and poured two more pots of water over the cooker, just to make sure the fire was out.

I came out of the house and sat on a bench in the neighbour's front garden. I was totally exhausted and worn out.

About fifteen minutes later the fire service arrived and asked me what happened.

Two of them went into the house while one of them stayed with me and made sure I was all right.

They checked the house out, and then they got into the fire engine and drove off. They did not even say goodbye or thanks to me.

I was so disappointed that day, not one of the fire men thanked me.

I slowly and painfully made my way back to Mary's house and made myself a cup of coffee.

I sat on the chair in the kitchen and I wondered what in the name of God just happened.

I finished my coffee and decided to have a mid morning nap.

Lana and I popped up on the camp bed and I quickly drifted into a light sleep.

Suddenly Lana started barking. I sat up and looked out the window.

I could see the neighbour walking up the drive way.

She knocked on the door I answered it.

She hugged me and smiled at me and said, "Thank you Tony and that's from the bottom of my heart."

I smiled back at her and said that's no bother girl I would do the same for anybody.

She then went back to her house.

I turned the T.V. on, and I propped myself up on some cushions. I watched total crap for the rest of the day.

Mary and the kids returned to the house at about four o clock.

I complemented Mary on her stunning new hair do. She hugged me and said, "Thanks Tony."

Mary then asked me how my day was. I then said you're not going to believe what happened.

I told her of the events of the morning.

She was flabbergasted amused and amazed at my fireman Sam antics. Then out of nowhere she said, "You should have left it burn."

Mary and the neighbour had being arguing since the very first day they moved into their new homes six months ago.

Basically the whole argument was about the chickens in the neighbour's garden, shouting their mouths off early every single daybreak.

Mary started to prepare dinner, and I started playing with the children. As usual Mary left out a roar and asked us to calm down a bit.

Ten minutes later Mary dished out ribs and cabbage.

Everybody went silent as we munched into and enjoyed our food.

When we all finished our dinner I cleaned the table and loaded the dishwasher for her.

Mary told the children to go to their bedrooms and do their home work. They did and the house fell silent.

I decided to have a soak in a salt water bath.

Mary ran the bath for me, and five minutes later I was up to my neck in salt water. I stayed in the bath for at least an hour, and I tried to soak away my upcoming surgery. It was impossible to stop thinking about Can-sir, because at this stage I felt it was written on the black board of my mind.

The kids were calling out to use the toilet. By now they were all ready for bed.

I tried to get out of the bath, and I found it was near impossible.

I called Mary in and without hesitation she helped me out of the bath. I struggled to dress myself.

I said good night to the kids, and I told Mary that I was exhausted and worn out. Mary said, "Tony go to bed for yourself and try to get some sleep."

I lay down on Mary's bed with my well travelled friend Kidney as I tried to pray myself to sleep.

Suddenly I realised I had not got my magical and mystical Rosary Beads with me.

I could genuinely feel myself panicking.

I called Mary and asked her had she seen them.

Mary said, "Tony your beads are in the sitting room on the window sill, I will get them for you."

Two minutes later Mary passed me my bunch of worn out precious beads. Mary left the bed room to go and watch T.V.

I wrapped my beads around my hand and I began to pray as time passed by my prayers turned into a form of meditation.

I found myself asking God for to help heal my wound, so I could be ready for my next major life threatening surgery. There was no doubt about my fear of what was laying ahead for me. Secretly I was bricking it but my prayer and meditation were helping to ease the strain of a pending death. I understood that night that

Heaven is not just open for heroes, its open to anybody who sincerely wants to get in.

I asked God to help me tap into my own wisdom and inner strength, and for some reason I think he helped me big time that night again.

I drifted off to sleep and suddenly it was early in the morning. I crept out of bed, and the sun wasn't even up, the house was silent.

I made some Star bucks and went out with Lana to see the sun rising and breaking through the clouds.

It was a magnificent fresh frosty winter morning. The trees in the distance were shimmering with light as the sun beams burst true their leaves. This can-sir seemed to have brought me closer to nature.

Suddenly the neighbour's chickens started their early morning routine.

Within thirty seconds Mary appeared at the back door.

By God she was very angry she left a few roars out and turned towards me and said, "It's your entire fault Tony."

I asked her why. She replied, "If you didn't put the fire out we all would have a bit of peace now."

I looked at Mary and tried to explain that I would do the same tomorrow for anybody.

I said to Mary stop don't go there.

Mary told me what to do with myself and it wasn't very nice.

Within five minutes I was in my car and heading towards Waterford City I switched my mobile off and threw it on the back seat. I felt myself getting tense and angrier as the miles passed by. By the time I got to Waterford my head was in an awful state.

I entered my house and switched my phone on, and I wasn't surprised to see seven abusive text messages from Mary, each one was progressively worse.

I switched my cell phone off again, and I tried to relax my mind.

But it was near impossible.

I made some star bucks coffee and a small Irish breakfast for myself.

Physically I was feeling o.k. but mentally I was definitely a bit disturbed that morning. I didn't want to turn my cell phone on; I felt it would bring more stress and tension upon me.

Suddenly my door bell rang.

Chapter Fourteen:

Grounding Myself Again

I answered the door and to my surprise it was my old work buddy Seamus.

I asked Seamus to try some star bucks coffee he just nodded his head at me.

I went to the kitchen and when I returned to the sitting room Seamus handed me a small bag of weed, and said, "Tony I heard about your troubles and I know the weed is used in other countries for some Can- Sir patients."

He slipped his hand into his pocket and pulled out a ready made joint. He handed it to me and said, "Get that into you boy, I will guarantee you all your troubles will be in the past."

He was right. Two puffs and I felt as high as the sky.

Suddenly I realised that my pain had diminished and most of my worries were temporarily on hold, and it felt damn good. As a matter of fact this was the best I felt since my first surgery.

Seamus and I chatted for at least an hour, and then Seamus asked me did I want to go for a spin in the country. It didn't take much persuading to get me into Seamus' van that day.

Seamus drove to a beach in West Waterford called Kilfarrisey; it's a small beach with two small islands a couple of hundred meters from the shore. My parents always brought us there when we were young children.

I always felt happy when I was there.

Seamus stayed in the van and I went for a walk on the beach. It was a very rough and windy day the sea was crashing violently on the shore line and the rain was belting down.

I sat on a big boulder close to the bottom of the cliffs.

I felt that there was something primal and nourishing about this place.

It felt like this was a place of personal empowerment and peace.

Suddenly I heard Seamus beeping the horn; I walked back up the beach and got back into the van.

Seamus passed me another joint of weed and said, "Get that into you man." I took a few puffs and I put it out. I felt a bit dizzy.

I asked Seamus was he capable to drive. He did not reply he just started laughing at me.

We drove down the coast road, and Seamus asked me did I want to go to Mount Mellary.

Instantly I replied yes. Seamus said, "No bother man we are on our way."

I sat back and enjoyed the spin.

Fifteen minutes later Seamus stopped the van on the side of the road. I asked him what's up.

He replied, "Come on Tony I want to show you something special."

We climbed over a gate and made our way to a small dense forest.

We entered the forest and within five minutes of walking, I was amazed and amused to see a grotto of the queen of peace nestled in among the forest.

Seamus knelt down at the grotto and said, "Tony this is a very special and holy place."

I knelt down beside him and I began to pray in my mind, suddenly the hairs on the back of my neck stood up like a dog getting ready for a fight.

I told Seamus about the hairs and he said, "Tony when ever I come here the same thing always happens to me when I start praying."

We stayed there in silence for about ten minutes.

125

Suddenly Seamus said, "Come on Tony we have an hour of driving to get to Mellary."

We made our way back to the van and continued on our mini spiritual holiday.

An hour later and we were in Mount Mellary.

Seamus stopped the van in a small sloped car park, and both of us made our way to the grotto.

Seamus had a bandage on his wrist he had damaged a tendon, while knocking down a wall with a sledge hammer a couple of days before.

He removed the bandage and showed me his wrist.

Every time he moved his fingers a big lump would appear just above his wrist, and when he straightened his fingers the lump would disappear, and he was also in a bit of pain. I asked him did he go to the doctor he just laughed at me and said, "My doctor is here."

I knew exactly what was up with his hand.

Three years ago I over stretched my hand in work, and the same thing happened to me. I went to the doctor he wrapped it up and said it would take six to eight weeks to fully heal ,and it did take six weeks.

Seamus walked over to a small well just in front of the grotto, and steeped his sore hand in the water for a couple of minutes.

He turned towards me and said, "O God Tony this is a very holy place."

I was deep in prayer so I just nodded back at him.

We eventually left the grotto and went to the grounds of the Abbey.

Seamus went off on his own wandering through the gardens, and I went into the Abbeys chapel and knelt down. I thanked the man above for just being here, and for every breath that I was taking.

This place seemed to strengthen my belief that some day I would be well again.

Twenty minutes later and Seamus entered the small chapel in the Abbey.

He came over to me and said, "Come on we are on our way."

I got up and we walked out together and jumped into the van. We drove the coast road home, and an hour and a half later we were back in my house.

I put the coffee on and Seamus went into the sitting room.

Five minutes later I handed him his coffee and he handed me another joint. I said I don't think I would be able for it right now. He said, "No problem buddy put it away with your bag for later."

He then had to go as his boss was texting him.

We gave each other a buddy hug and he left my house. The last thing he said to me was, "Call out tomorrow buddy."

By now I was hungry so I made myself some scrambled egg and toast. I sat in the sitting room and watched the six o clock news, as I munched away at my food. When I was finished I switched my cell phone on and all as I heard was bleep-bleep-bleep. I got three text messages from Mary.

The first one read where are you.

The second one; who are you with.

And the third one read; I am sorry.

I rang Mary and we calmly chatted for a while.

Mary was insisting that I drive down to her, and I was adamant to stay in my home with my son for the night.

I told Mary I needed some time to sort my head out, and to prepare for my second life threatening surgery, that was only a couple of weeks away.

Mary wasn't too happy with me staying in Waterford.

I told her that I would ring her first thing in the morning and we hung up.

I had been with her for four years and this was not the first time that tension and temper tantrums had appeared in our relationship.

I phoned my son Shane and told him I was up in my house. I asked him did he want to come up. Shane replied, "No dad I am playing indoor soccer tonight." I said ok so love you Shane and we hung up.

I then lit a big fire and turned the emersion on for a salt bath.

Twenty minutes later and I was in the bath trying to soak my worries and trouble and pains away.

I finished my bath and I made a great effort to get out, and put my P jays on. I then sat down in the sitting room, and started to watch the television. I was comfortable and at peace with my self and the world.

It got late so I went to bed and said my prayers, and snuggled into kidney and drifted off to sleep.

I got out of bed at seven the next morning.

I made some Star Bucks and lit the fire.

I sat back on the arm chair and began to watch the early morning T.V. shows.

I was starting to get bored and agitated. I switched my phone on and as soon as I did it started to ring.

I looked at the number and answered. It was my buddy Seamus, he asked me how I was feeling. I told him I was feeling confused agitated and bored.

He told me to snap out of it and start living in the here and now.

He asked me could he call up for a chat. He told me that he had something to show me. I said see you in ten minutes and we hung up.

I put some more coffee on just as Seamus arrived at my front door.

The first thing out of his mouth was, "Tony look at my hand." He held his hand out and bent his fingers towards the ground and flexed them up again.

He and I were totally amazed and amused.

Seamus hand showed no sign of injury.

We both realised that morning that miracles are real and they do happen. Even if they are only small ones.

Seamus had his coffee and we chatted for a while, and then he wished me well and the last thing he said to me was, "Tony God is good to those who are good to others." As he left my house my spirit was in good form.

I phoned Mary and told her I wanted to stay in Waterford for a few more days.

I explained to her that this was probably the last chance I would possibly get to hang out with my family and friends.

With a small bit of anger in her voice she accepted this and let it go.

I spent the next week and a half wandering between Waterford and Wexford. Driving up and down every second day. As I drove I prayed constantly, and some how this switched my mind away from the pending surgery, and my possible plausible death.

Being on the country road so much my pain was starting to creep back in to my wound.

I ignored it and told myself to be strong and accept it.

And I did. For every night that I stayed in my house I dipped into my bag of weed, and to tell the truth as soon as I was stoned, I did not give a shit about can-sir or surgeries or pain or dying. It seemed like the weed was blocking my mind from all negative thoughts, feelings and emotions.

As they say time waits for no man. The days passed quickly by and suddenly I realised it was Wednesday evening, two days before my next life threatening surgery.

Mary the kids and I were all in the sitting room watching the movie Buzz Light Year, and suddenly my phone rang.

I quickly left the room and answered it.

It was Theresa my earthly angel, she phoned to tell me she had arranged the hotel again for Mary. Theresa phoned me because she did not want to talk to Mary. They really did not get on well together while we were in America.

She wished me good health and said, "Tony most of the people in the factory are lighting candles and praying for you to survive." I thanked her and asked her to thank all them one by one for their kindness.

I went back to the sitting room. As soon as I entered Mary asked me "Who was on the phone."

I told her it was Theresa. Mary asked me what she wanted. I told her Theresa arranged the hotel in Dublin.

Mary replied and said, "Why didn't she ring me?

I quickly said your guess is as good as mine.

I left the sitting room and went to the kitchen Lana came with me. I walked out the back door and went to the Grotto, and sat on the bench.

I remember so clearly that night asking God to help me on this long and daunting safari through can-sir.

Sudden I burst out crying, and it felt like I was drowning in my own tears. I had to tell myself to stop acting like a baby.

I stayed there for at least a half an hour with Lana's head on my lap. My feelings that evening were anger, denial, and last of all I felt like I was bargaining with the all mighty for my life.

When I returned to the house the children were in bed. Mary was in the front porch smoking a cigarette.

I sensed she was not in a good mood, so I asked her what's up. Instantly she started on about the cheek of Theresa ringing me instead of her.

I asked her to let it go and she replied in a smart tone "Why should I!"

I told her to cop on and try to look at things from my prospective for a moment.

She smiled at me and said, "Tony I suppose you're right."

Mary had a habit of making Mountains out of mole hills, and this always pissed me off, more so now in my illness than before my illness.

I told her I felt knackered and I needed sleep.

We locked the house up, and Mary went to her bedroom to watch some television.

I went to my camp bed and lay down, and I began to prey. I realised that night that I was praying hard for my life. I suddenly understood that counting on humans I could never win. As usual Lana woke me up before dawn. I got dressed and opened the front door, Lana bolted out. I grabbed her lead and followed her.

She did her business and I put her lead on her. We strolled to the grotto near the old railway track.

I said a small few meaningful prayers and I wondered was I seeking fools gold. We walked slowly back to the house, and as I did I wondered who is to blame. On the way back Lana stuck to my right side. I repeatedly pulled her to the left and she kept looking at me and returning to my right side. I knew she sensed something was wrong with my right side this time.

Lana and I arrived back at the house at about half past eight.

Mary and the kids were heading to school. I waved them off, and I made myself some star bucks.

I sat in the bird garden and I tried to keep fear away from my brain, but it was near impossible.

It seemed like I was looking at my life without being in it. For some strange reason I understood that death doesn't like to be cheated.

I wondered was it possible to survive, and forge a new future for myself.

When I look back at this drama in my life, I wonder was this Gods way of slowing me down.

Mary returned to the house and asked me to go shopping with her. Instantly I said yes. I would have done anything that day to keep my mind away from what lay ahead for me.

An hour or so later Mary and I were in the centre of Wexford town.

I bought a pair of jeans and an Aran jumper, and two track suits to wear when I was released from hospital.

We returned to the house at about one o clock.

I tried to settle my mind but it was near impossible.

Fear anger and frustration were creeping in as the time ticked by. I decided to drive to Waterford to; possibly say my last goodbyes to family and friends. Mary wasn't too happy with my decision but she had no choice.

As I drove towards Waterford my negative thoughts started too recede.

I visited friends first and than family.

I collected Shane and we drove to my house.

We spent a couple of precious hours together, and then Shane's mum and Sister Elaine my precious step daughter collected him. I stood at the front door and waved them off. Elaine and Shane blew a kisses at me as they drove off.

I welled up with sadness for there was a big possibility that I would never see them again.

I lit the fire to heat the water, and twenty minutes later I popped into a salt bath and tried to unwind my mind.

I finished my bath and sat myself down by the big roaring fire.

I switched the television on and to my horror the medical programme E.R. was on. I turned the television off and I put some instrumental music on. I tried to relax but it was virtually impossible.

I was starting to feel very down and depressed.

I wondered to myself was this my last few day on earth.

Suddenly my phone rang. I answered it and it was my buddy Seamus. He asked me was I still in Waterford.

I said yes. Seamus said, "Tony do you need anything."

I replied and said no thanks buddy.

Seamus said, "No bother Tony I am on my way up to you, see you in ten minutes."

Seamus arrived and I made him some coffee.

When I returned to the sitting room he handed me a big fat joint of pure weed, but he never told me it was pure with no tobacco in it.

I lit it and took a couple of puffs and instantly I was stoned beyond belief.

Seamus looked at me and burst out laughing.

I asked him what's so funny. Seamus replied and said, "Tony your eyes are like pee holes in the snow."

I stood up and looked in the mirror, and I agreed with his observation and burst out laughing. He stayed with me and helped me pack my hospital sports kit.

We continually laughed and took the piss out of each other for the next hour.

Seamus's phone beeped he looked at it and said, "Tony I got to go the boss wants me home."

He shuck my hand and then he said in a serious tone, "You'll be all right, Tony God is good to those who are good, take care of yourself Tony and I'll see you soon." I replied and said please God and his blessed mother.

It was nine o clock when Seamus left my home.

I returned to the sitting room and sat down on the couch.

I rang Mary and told her that I was in no state to drive.

She asked me why.

I told her about my evening with my friend.

I expected her to be angry towards me but this time I was wrong.

Mary told me that she had arranged for the kids to be picked up from the school for the next day, and their nanny and aunties were going to look after them while we were in Dublin.

Mary asked me to go to bed and get some sleep, and she said, "Don't forget to set your alarm Tony."

I blew a kiss down the phone and said, god bless and hung up.

I picked up what was left of the joint and vigorously hogged it in to me.

I bounced and bopped my way to my bedroom, and knelt down beside the bed and said my prayers. I then set my alarm for five A.M.

As soon as my head hit the pillow I began to pray from my heart and soul. I wondered how I could thank the almighty for his help for getting me this far. It seemed like my prayer and confidence in the lord was leading me towards a healthful way of thinking. That night during my prayers I realised that every breath is a blessing, and if I wanted to survive I must have a healthy mind and a positive outlook.

As I lay there I felt like God was helping me through my troubles and anxieties.

That night it felt like I was beginning to disarm all my internal hostility, and I was removing mental obstacles from my path.

My thoughts deepened, and I thought that this sorrow that I was enduring must have something deeper in it. It must penetrate into my sole and it must transform its self into action. That night I felt like a small bit of hope was shining in my heart and spirit. I drifted of into a soft peaceful sleep.

Suddenly the alarm beeped. As my eyes opened a wave of deep intense fear ran true my whole body and mind. I felt semi paralysed in the bed. That morning with great difficulty I shuffled my self out of bed.

I had a bath and dressed myself and made some Star Bucks coffee. As soon as the coffee was in me, my spirit began to rise

This was the morning of the day of my second big surgery and by now I felt mentally and physical ready for death or survival.

I tried to potter around my house for a couple of hours, praying as I did my chores. I was in a good mood. I found this a bit strange considering the day that I had ahead of me.

I put my bits and pieces in my car, and I locked up my house. It was eight in the morning and I drove off to Mary's house. There was little traffic on the roads so I made good time. I prayed as I drove all the way to county Wexford.

Chapter Fifteen:
Fearful Return

I arrived at Mary's house at about ten past nine.

As usual Lana came to greet me.

I walked into the house and Mary and the children were having their breakfast.

I was so hungry looking at them eating; my tummy was rumbling big time so I had to leave the kitchen.

I walked to the grotto in the garden and sat on the bench, and I wondered was this the end of days for me. I began to cry as my thoughts deepened. I wondered was I spiritually fit to tackle the challenge ahead.

I knew that if I wanted to live I would have to draw energy and strength from the universe above.

Suddenly Mary called me from the kitchen window.

I returned to the house and hugged the children, and then Mary drove them to school. Secretly I wondered would I ever see them all again.

Mary came back a half hour later and said, "Tony I forgot about Lana." She phoned the children's dad and asked him to collect Lana, he said no bother consider it done.

Mary put Lana in the shed and locked up her house.

She put her bags in the boot of my car, and that was it we were on the road heading for the Mater hospital in Dublin again.

Mary asked me did I confirm my bed. I said Mary that was a million miles away from my mind.

She rang the bed management team and all was sorted in a matter of minutes.

When she hung up she said, "Tony you're not going to believe this, its Saint Anthony's ward and its bed number one again."

This was the same bed that I was in a month earlier.

After three hours of driving on the pot hole knackered roads of Ireland, we arrived at the hotel and Mary checked us in.

We went to our room and instantly I lay down for a rest.

She unpacked her bags as I tried to quash my thoughts and deepest fears. Mary went for a bite to eat, and I just lay there with Kidney in my arms wondering and worrying and trying to resolve my fear.

Mary returned at one o clock and said, "Are you ready to go Tony."

I replied will I ever be ready. She smiled at me and said, "Come on or we'll be late."

We made our way to the under ground car park.

We got in my car, and I drove the short distance straight to the Mater hospital long term car park.

I secretly wanted to turn the car around and go home, and take my chances with time.

Mentally I struggled to get out of the car. It felt like my body was shutting down.

I grabbed Kidney and my small hospital sports kit.

I locked the car, and Mary and I made our way to the reception area of the Mater hospital.

I checked in and we proceeded to Saint Anthony's ward. As we walked my silly mind was throwing up some awful disturbing scenarios. Stuff like was this my green mile. Will I get out of here?

And if so would I be disabled and dysfunctional.

When we arrived at the ward we were welcomed by the sister of the ward.

She escorted me to my bed and asked me to put my P.jays on.

Mary pulled the curtains around the bed, and I undressed and put my new commando P.jays on. I nervously sat on the bed.

Mary pulled the curtains open, and as she did I felt my heart rate increasing. Within sixty seconds it felt like my heart was going to pop out of my chest. By this stage all of my positive thoughts were depleted.

This was the first time that I truly understood the concept fight or flight.

I told Mary I was going to the toilet, and I made my way out of the ward and did my pe pe. Because it was the old part of the hospital the toilets for the ward were out in the main hallway.

Suddenly a terrifying fear invaded my whole body and mind, and possibly my spirit as well.

Without being fully aware of my actions, I suddenly found myself bolting from the hospital, just like a rabbit bolting from his burrow.

I slowly walked the perimeter of the hospital.

On my short journey I noticed mount Joy prison. It was straight opposite the accident and emergency unit at the back end of the hospital. I stopped walking and lit a cigarette. I stared at the prison and wondered were they better off than me, and my conclusion that day was yes they were.

I wandered on with fear in my mind, and made my way to the front new part of the hospital. As I was walking along I noticed a poor destitute person sitting on the ground with a begging hat by his side.

When I got close to him he asked me for some spare change. Shit I was in my P.jays and I had no money on me.

I told him I had no money on me, so I offered him a cigarette instead. I had two cigarettes left and I gave him one. I lit the other one and asked him could I sit with him for a while. He answered and said, "Please do sir."

As we chatted a flashy Mercedes Bens pulled up by the kerb.

A well dressed man got out and walked to the parking ticket machine and put his money in it.

Suddenly the man sitting by me asked the well dressed man for some change.

The well dressed man just looked at us and started to walk away. The poor man with me said, "Thanks any way sir and God bless you sir."

Suddenly the well dressed man spun around, and reached into his pocket and wipe out five euro. He smiled and gently placed it in the poor mans hat. He then turned on his heels and walked on.

The poor man and I looked at each other in recognition of a mini miracle.

I built up the courage and asked him his name he said, "My name is Anthony."

Instantly the hairs stood up on the back of my neck and shoulders. I told him my name and all about Saint Anthony's ward.

We were both amazed and amused. He then said, "There is something special about you Anthony."

I asked him what brought him to this point in his life.

He told me that his partner died three weeks ago from a lethal dose of bad heroin in his flat, and he could not face going back to the flat that she died in.

I felt so sorry for this man, and I think he felt sorry for me.

Suddenly two big hospital security guards appeared on the scene. One of them asked me my name, as soon as I told them my name; the other one grabbed my arm and said in a thick ignorant voice, "Mister Power the doctors are waiting on you."

I told him to remove his hand or the doctors will be waiting on him. He removed his hand instantly.

Suddenly my new found friend stood up and said lads take it easy. I told the security guards to go and have a ---- for them selves, and I will come back when I am good and ready.

The smallest one of them said, "Ok Mister Power we will wait at the main door for you, and try not leave it too long or your surgery will be cancelled."

I replied and said no bother lads.

Talk to me nice and I will be nice back to ye.

Maybe I was a bit overboard and outspoken, but nobody has the right to put their hands on anybody else.

I sat back down and Anthony said, "For a small and sick man to stand up to those clowns must mean you're strong on the inside."

Anthony asked me could he walk with me to the main door. I said it would be a pleasure sir.

Anthony helped me get up off the pavement, and we walked slowly towards the main door. While we were walking Anthony asked two young pretty foreign girls for a cigarette. One of them smiled at us and handed Anthony the packet and said keep them. He thanked them, and then we went straight to the smoking area just outside the main entrance of the hospital.

I smoked my last cigarette and Anthony walked with me to the main door. I shook his hand and we wished each other good health and then we parted.

I entered the main door and Beavis and Butthead were waiting for me, with a wheel chair by their side.

I got an uncontrollable bout of laughter as I sped my pace up and passed them by.

I entered Saint Anthony's ward with the two security guards in tow. As soon as I entered Mister Murphy pointed at my bed and said, "Get in now Tony."

I lay down and Mister Murphy put his hands on my arm, and stared at me and said, "Tony you're an awkward patient."

I just nodded in acceptance of his statement.

He also told me that this surgery was a matter of life and death, and if it wasn't preformed immediately I would be dead within two weeks.

He practically scared the breath out of my lungs.

He also said, "Tony if you survive you will probably have a tube coming from your chest, so we can hook you up to a dialysis machine."

I thought to myself I would be better off dead.

Then he gave me two tablets and said, "Swallow."

I asked him what they were and he replied "Anxicalm."

He passed me a glass of water from my locker and I swallowed the two tablets, and then he said, "I will see you when you come round after surgery." He then left the ward in a wicked hurry.

Mary held my hand as I drifted off into a semi conscious state of mind.

Soon my taxi driver arrived with his pretty little chariot.

As dopey as I was, I still managed to get in the wheel chair under my own steam.

On my way to the operating room I began to think I must face up to the fear of my surgery.

We arrived at the pre op room and I said to Mary if I don't see you later on, I will see you in heaven.

She burst out crying as I was wheeled in through the doors.

I laid there nervously waiting.

Suddenly a small dark skinned bald man with round glasses approached me. He introduced himself and said,

"I am your anaesthetist and I need to ask you a few routine questions about your medical history."

I answered them to the best of my memories ability.

Suddenly he asked me to show him my arms.

I unclenched my arms and moved them above the bed sheet.

He looked at me and said what's in your hand.

I unclenched my fist, and my bunches of Rosary Beads were revealed.

He looked at me and said in an Indian voice, "Mister Power you can't have them in here."

I told him if the beads go I go with them.

"No no no" he said.

I looked at him face on, and said yes yes yes.

He disappeared and returned a couple of minutes later with Mister Murphy by his side.

Mister Murphy put out his hand, as he did he asked me were they the same beads as before. I gave him my beads and said yes boss. He disappeared and returned a couple of minutes later.

He told me to move my head up.

I did and he gently placed my iodine stained Beads around my neck. He knew the routine no beads no surgery.

I was thrilled to bits and now I was happy to proceed.

Mister Murphy lowered his head towards mine and said, "Tony you're an awful trouble maker but they're the ones that nearly always get well again."

My actions and his words infused me with a bit of hope.

The anaesthetist proceeded to hook me up to what looked like a futuristic space age machines.

For a brief moment I felt scared and isolated.

Gandhi abruptly punctured my right arm and pumped in some chemicals.

He placed a mask over my nose and mouth and said, "Count to ten."

I tried to count but I only made it to five and that was all I remember.

Six or seven hours later my eyes slowly opened but it seemed like my brain was still asleep.

I slowly scanned the room and this effort delapated the small bit of strength that I had left in reserve.

I vaguely remember somebody rubbing water on my lips.

I tried to speak but it wasn't happening.

I tried to open my eyes again but it was impossible.

I tried to listen but all sounds seemed muttered and muddled up.

I was told afterwards that I remained in this state for three days, only waking up to vomit.

On the third day I was aware that somebody was standing over my bed praying. I was also feeling mind blowing pain from my surgery site.

I used all my last bit of inner strength and courage to open my eyes.

I was shocked beyond belief to see a priest standing their administering me the last rights. Tears flowed like never before.

I thought this is it; I am on my way to the other world, and I wondered was my journey going to be up or down.

The priest anointed me with his magic bottle of holy oil and wished me well and left my bed side.

I lay their waiting for that horrific moment to come but thank God and his Blessed Mother it never did.

I assessed my pain and I noted it at nine out of ten.

My tummy and scars felt like they were going to explode at any moment, but yet I was still alive, and I realised I had the remotest chance of survival.

Suddenly a black male nurse was at my bed side.

He gently placed his hand on mine and told me his name was Israel, and he was from South Africa.

I sensed a sense of peace and comfort and serenity coming from this man, and I never felt any thing like it in my whole life.

He asked me to point to where the pain felt the strongest.

I pointed to my tummy and remained silent.

He walked to his station and I could see his hands fumbling around in a narrow cabinet.

He returned and gave me a small plastic see through cup and the contents looked like Guinness.

I swigged this vile concoction down, and Israel sat with me and chatted about his home land and his faith for at least fifteen minutes.

By now my tummy was rumbling it was a small bit embarrassing, for I knew the whole ward was aware of it.

Without any effort wind broke from behind.

Now I was truly mortified.

Israel called another male nurse over and he introduced himself in the gayest of voice as Gavin from Naven. They both began to detach me from the mesh of wires and tubes inserted in my body.

Israel moved my legs over the side of the bed.

I placed my feet on the ground.

I tried to stand up but my legs had not got the strength to support my body.

Israel and Gavin placed their arms under my shoulders and with great effort and difficulty they shuffled me out of the ward and we entered the toilet.

Isreal pulled my P.jays down and they both sat me down on the toilet, Gavin said, "Fire away to your hearts content."

Isreal said, "Tony we will be outside the door and when you're finished don't try to get up."

After a couple of minutes an explosion occurred.

I cleaned myself as best as I could.

I then grabbed on to the wash hand basin and with all my strength I pulled myself upright.

I looked in the mirror and to my horror I looked and felt like I was not far away from death. I never felt so sick or close to death in my whole life. I was terrified I looked in the mirror again as tears streamed past my cheeks, and I sincerely asked God to heal me or take me home.

Suddenly my weak and weary legs collapsed.

I fell through the unlocked door and Israel broke my fall.

Unfortunately I had knocked Israel to the ground and I landed on top of him.

My P.jays were still down around my ankles and the scene looked like something that it wasn't.

We all burst out in hysterical laughter.

Gavin put his arm under mine and pulled me upright, and with one hand held me there, and with the other one he quickly pulled my p jays up.

Israel was still on the ground in hysterics.

When he got up and eventually controlled his laughing, he said, "That was the funniest thing that has ever happened to him in his whole life."

I said lads it's funny but it has probably scarred me mentally for the rest of my life. The boys returned me to the ward and put me on the bed, and hooked me back up to the gadgets and gismos that surrounded my bed.

Between my last rights, and my encounter with Israel and Gavin my spirit and body had increased its strength and power, and I felt like living again.

I really believe that the fun and laughter and humour of that morning began the healing process within me.

The two boys left my bed as they were still giggling.
I grabbed my beads and began to pray and give thanks.
Suddenly I remembered what Mister Murphy had said to me a few minutes before my second surgery.
I reached my hand up to my chest and frantically searched for a tube of some sort.

I really can't explain how I felt when I didn't find one.
The only thing I can say about that moment is that I naturally felt higher than high. I asked my God to help me direct my thinking, and I asked him to diminish all self pity within me.

I started to analyse things in my head. I looked over the side of my bed and saw that my pe bag was three quarters full.

I saw this as an indication that the four fifths of my last kidney was working; and working well.
The events of the morning took its toll on me.
I was very tired but I was also very happy just to be breathing.
I started to drift off to sleep with my polar bear in my arms.
Suddenly I felt my bear friend being removed from my arms.
I opened my eyes and Mister Murphy was standing there with a grin on his face.
He said, "Tony you're a remarkable man."
I asked him what he meant.
He told me that when he opened me for surgery he froze my kidney, and sliced away the bad part, and even before he stitched my kidney back, it was producing urine.
He then left and as he did he said, "See you tomorrow Tony."
Now I felt like I had a million billion reasons to appreciate and value what was left of my life.
I felt like I got much more than I ever hoped and dreamed and prayed for.
A short while later Mary arrived at my bed.
I could sense she was in bad form.

I asked her what the problem was.

She snapped at me and said "You."

Mary accused me of flirting with the nurses on the ward.

Soon our conversation elevated to an argument.

Mary told me what to do with myself, and I abruptly returned the compliment.

Mary then left the ward, and I was left lying there speechless and very upset and down in myself. The whole atmosphere of the ward had changed for the worst.

Israel slowly wandered over to me and asked me what that was all about.

I told him that Mary was a very jealous person, and if she wasn't the centre of attention all hell would break loose.

I tried to quieten my mind but it was near impossible.

Out of nowhere, I suddenly needed to be on my own.

I asked Israel to pull the curtains and leave me alone.

He did and I presume he returned to his station.

As I lay there I found myself sinking into a deep depressive state of mind.

That day it seamed like my mind was trapped between reality and unreality.

The small bit of serenity left in me was being attacked by my morbid senseless thoughts.

I tucked into Kidney and began to pray with my knotted up bundle of beads clenched tightly in my hand.

My prayer was interrupted by a small portly Irish demanding nurse. I asked her to leave me alone she didn't reply she just untangled some tubes and left.

Over the next two days everybody that had approached me got the cold shoulder from me. Except for a middle aged cleaning lady with a Northern Ireland accent.

She brought me my food, and arranged my pain killers, and emptied my pe bag regularly.

Every time she approached me I felt an angelic presence emanating from her. She wore a pink uniform and always did more than her duties for me.

Suddenly my phone beeped. I picked it up and looked at the number and lo and behold it was Mary. I read the message and basically it was an apology.

I texted her and asked her where she was.

Mary texted back, and her message read, "At home will talk tomorrow." I switched the phone off and placed it on my locker.

I must have drifted off to sleep because the next thing I remember was Mister Murphy waking me up.

Immediately he said, "Tony it's your lucky day."

I asked him why.

He answered me in a cheerful voice and said, "Tony if your bloods are good I will disconnect you from every thing."

He insisted that I increase my water intake to at least three litres a day, and told me that if I didn't, it would diminish my chances of going home soon.

I asked him what he meant by soon, and he answered and said, "Three or four days, Tony it depends on you."

He left my bed side and disappeared out of the ward.

He left me with the word home repeating in my brain.

The more I repeated the word (home) the more I felt my spirits being lifted. It's amazing how in an instant one word brought me from rock bottom to sky high.

Time passed by and soon my blood sucker was by my side again.

I willingly gave her my arm and shut my eyes tightly, and waited for the pain of my puncture.

She inserted her long pointy weapon and drew blood from my arm.

The nurse put a small plaster over my needle wound and said, "Thank you Mister Power" as she moved on to the next victim. I turned my head and asked her how long would the results take.

She turned her head towards me and said, "At least an hour Mister Power."

I tried to occupy myself with some reading but it was virtually impossible. My mind kept wondering to the front door and back again.

Eventually Israel and Gavin came to my bed side, and Israel said, "Tony your bloods are normal and your Creatine level is one hundred and twenty two."

I asked him to excuse my ignorance, and what the Creatine level meant.

He told me it's the level of function in the kidneys.
I asked him what the proper level should be.
He smiled at me and said, "One two two."
Instantly the level of happiness increased within me.
I felt all is well and I would only get stronger as the days passed by. Israel disconnected my wires and tubes, and the last thing for him to do was to remove the pipe from my manhood.

Gavin held my hand tightly and Israel proceeded to do his job in a dignified professional manner.

I tightly closed my eyes, and Israel quickly removed my temporary toilet, as he did I felt a blast of enormous pain in my we man for a couple of seconds.

This pain felt like the mother of all pains, but thank God it disappeared as quickly as it had arrived.

I asked Israel would it be possible to get some fresh air. He looked at me and said, "Tony your legs won't carry you". I answered him and said lets give it a go anyway.

With all the strength that was left in my body, I moved my legs to the side of the bed.

Gavin held on to me as I placed my feet on the ground.

I stood upright and as soon as I did I was forced to accept the reality of my situation.

I was temporarily semi paralysed.

Gavin said, "Tony I have a good idea" and turned on his heels and left the ward.

A couple of minutes later he returned with what looked like a wheel chair. I was a bit stunned because it was a potty on wheels.

Israel looked at Gavin and said, "Are you for real."
Gavin replied, "It's up to Tony."
As they waited for my answer my head quickly went into overdrive.
After a brief moment of contemplation I answered and said, lads anyway out of here is better than being rolled out in a coffin.

Without hesitation they both put me into my potty chair, and they wheeled me to the front door's of the hospital.
As soon as the doors opened I took a deep breath of air, and at that moment, I truly believed that my inner healing had begun.

I quickly scanned my surroundings and I noticed people of all sorts and all ailments standing there smoking.
I asked an elderly gentle man for a cigarette, he passed me two cigarettes and I thanked him.

Israel looked at me and said, "Tony this is not on."
I looked back at him and said, your right and I told him that there was no point in smoking unless I had a coffee.
Gavin disappeared and shortly returned with coffee for us all.

I lit my first cigarette and sipped my coffee.
I felt deep inside that I was treating myself after all I had being through. I also felt that this ritual was helping me to return to normality and reality as quick as possible.

I was then returned to Saint Anthony's ward. The lads placed me back in my bed and they returned to their station.
Five minutes later Gavin returned and passed me the ward phone, I said hello and Mary answered me.
She asked me how I was feeling and in the same breath, why my cell phone was turned off.
I told her I was feeling o. k. and the cell phone thing slipped my mind.

We spoke for at least ten minutes, and then Mary told me she had a bad dose of the flu.

I felt disappointed because I hoped that she would come back to the hospital soon.

We blew kisses down the line and we both hung up.

I was tired after my first adventure to the outside, so I lay there and drifted into a prayer induced sleep.

A couple of hours later I woke to the sound of the squeaky wheels of the medication trolley.

A small kind Pilipino nurse handed me two morphine pain killers.

I swallowed them with a glass of water and I scrunched my beads tightly in my hand, and suddenly the next day had arrived.

I looked at the time; it was half past six in the morning.

The place was in an eerie silence.

I quickly focused and I assessed the ability of the mobility of my legs.

To my enjoyment and amazement they felt ten times better than yesterday. I silently and gently placed my feet on the floor, and with a slight effort I stood upright.

I slowly and silently made my way out of the ward without being noticed. I headed for the toilet staying close to the wall as I walked on.

I made it there and back again without any major incident.

Twenty minutes later my gourmet breakfast was served up.

I finished it before the lady had served it to the other people in the ward. As she walked towards the door I called her over to me, and asked her was there any seconds.

She smiled at me and popped another portion of scrambled egg and toast, and more coffee on my bed tray.

It went down like water off a ducks back.

I had no sooner finished when Mister Murphy appeared with a young pretty lady,

And two well dressed young men.

He plucked my chart from the end of my bed, and he spent a couple of minutes assessing it. He handed my chart to the young lady, and told his small team of interns that I had a radical nefrectamy last month and he said, "last week we preformed a partial nefrectamy."

He sat on my bed and said, "Tony I saw you yesterday sitting in a commode wheel chair smoking a cigarette, and I presume you had a cup of coffee in your hand."

I answered with one word, and that was guilty.

He said, "I just walked on and burst out laughing to myself."

He looked at me and said, "Tony how are you feeling."

I told him honestly it feels brilliant to be alive.

He asked me about my pain, and I told him it's about four out of ten, and it's bearable without any pain killers at the moment.

He told me to keep up the good work.

He looked at me and said, "Tony it looks like you'll be home in three or four days." I asked him could I go for a breath of fresh air.

He told me to stand up on one leg for one minute.

I instantly flung my legs over the side of the bed and stood up on my left leg, and with courage and deep inner strength I held that pose until he told me to stop.

He held my hand as I sat down on the bed and said, "Tony I am going to sign you up for the Dublin City marathon or maybe even river dance."

I thanked him from the bottom of my heart, and he replied, "God bless see you tomorrow Tony."

He than moved on to his next patient, and I lay back down for ten minutes rest and recovery.

As soon as Mister Murphy left the ward I got out of bed and put my slippers on, and I made my merry way to the old entrance of the hospital. The automatic doors slid open. I walked out and instantly took a deep breath. I felt like Nelson Mandela being freed from prison.

I sat down on the steps and propped my back up against a pillar. I looked up at the deep blue winter sky, and I thanked the creator for enlightening my awareness of my inner strength and hope.

Eventually I stood up and I walked to the bottom of the steps, and with a Daffy Duck stride I walked from the old entrance to the new entrance a distance of about two hundred meters. I was proud of myself but I was very tired and weary.

I sat down on a bench in the smokers shack and asked a sad looking middle aged lady for a cigarette.

She passed me one, as she wiped the tears from her eyes.

I felt compelled to ask her was she all right, and I did.

She told me that the doctors were going to remove her womb at eight the next morning.

I could feel and see that she was stressed out of her head and afraid.

I asked her was there any anybody with her, she said, "No."

Then I asked her was anybody coming tomorrow, to my horror she answered no, as the tears streamed down her face.

With out thinking I said I will be here for you tomorrow, and I will come and visit you as soon as you're back in your ward after surgery. I sensed a small uplift in her mood by my offer, and she accepted it. We finished our smokes and I walked her slowly back to her ward.

As we walked on she asked me what I was doing here.

I gave her a brief description of my medical history.

We stopped walking and she looked at me and said, "God bless you young man."

I walked her to her bed and we sat and chatted for a good half hour.

I wished her well and as I left I blew her a kiss, and her eyes lit up instantly.

I gently walked back to my ward, and as I did pain started to show its ugly head again. By the time I got to my bed I was barely able to walk. I lay down and Gavin approached me and said, "Tony you don't look too well."

I told him that I think I done too much too soon.

He agreed with me and asked me did I want any pain killers.

I just nodded and closed my eyes.

A few minutes later Gavin returned he said, "Open wide." I did and he popped two tablets in my mouth.

I placed Kidney under my head, and snuggled into him and I drifted off to sleep with my magic beads wrapped around my wrist.

When I eventually woke up I instantly looked at my watch. It was eight thirty and the supper lady was doing her rounds. This totally confused me because time for supper was usually five thirty.

I looked towards the Nurses station, and I could see and hear in the distance, Israel and Gavin balling with laughter. Suddenly I realised I had been done. One of them had reset my watch while I was sleeping.

Gavin approached my bed, and while still grinning he apologised for his prank.

I accepted his apology with laughter.

The tea lady gave me omelette tomato and toast, and I really enjoyed it. I asked for seconds and I was told that there is no more.

Isreal said, "Tony I will get you fish and chips as soon as the ward quietens down." I thanked him and he returned to his station.

As I lay there I suddenly realised that all pain had left my body, and I was feeling normal again.

An hour later Isreal and Gavin entered my cubicle, and drew the curtains.

Isreal passed out the food and we all munched to our hearts content.

Gavin returned to his station, and Isreal stayed with me and we began to chat.

I gave Isreal a brief account of my life.

Then it was his turn. Some of the things that he told me literally upset my insides.

He told me he was beaten up and whipped, by another tribe, and left for dead in the street in front of his mother's home.

He removed his top and showed me his whip lashed scars.

Shit they were all over his upper body. At that moment my scars were insignificant.

He placed his top back on and said, "Tony I survived through my ordeal with the power of Jesus Christ by my side."

It saddened and sickened me to think that human beings could do this to others, under the disguise of religion, land, or culture.

His shift was coming to an end, and he asked me could we pray together.

I placed my beads in my hand and placed my hands together, and Isreal began to pray but his prayers were of a different manner.

He thanked god for his life, and he asked god for help to make my life flourish. He was the happiest person that I had ever met in my whole existence on this planet. When we finished preying we shuck hands.

He then left the ward, and I was left to ponder on our deep conversation.

I drifted off to sleep and lo and behold my alarm clock breakfast trolley woke me up.

I felt some pain but not enough to justify more morphine.

I was served a small egg and toast which did nothing for my hunger.

Suddenly my mind flashed back to yesterday, and to the promise I had made to the lady.

I got out of bed and I quickly made my way to the ladies ward.

I was stopped at the entrance by a small dark haired petite nurse.

I asked her about the lady, and she told me that she had just left for surgery.

The nurse asked me was I related to her. I said no and told her and that I met the lady yesterday for the first time.

I told the nurse that I had arranged to meet up with the lady before her surgery.

The nurse looked at me and said, "Would you please come back at around eleven o clock." She also told me that she knew of the lady and of her dilemma.

I said God bless and within ten minutes I was back in my bed taking things easy.

Within minutes of arriving my vampire was sucking blood again.

An hour or so passed by and Mister Murphy came to my bed side, and in a not so nice tone asked me where I had been.

I told him about my mini adventure.

He looked at me and in a very nice tone said, "Are you a Good Samaritan." I just nodded at him.

He picked my charts up and said, "Tony you're going home tomorrow." I felt ecstatic and overjoyed and delighted.

He encouraged me to finish my mini adventure, and wished me well as he left the ward.

As soon as he vanished I called one of the day nurses over, and asked her to source me a golden chariot with indicators. She roared out laughing and said, "Ill do my very best."

Ten minutes later I was in my hand powered chariot powering my way to the middle aged lady's ward.

I entered the ward and went straight to the lady's bed.

She was still out cold from her anaesthetic.

Out of nowhere a small nun with a bunch of flowers in her hands appeared by the wheel chair.

She smiled at me and said, "Are you family." I said no.

Suddenly the lady began to wake up. With dopey eyes she smiled at the Nun and me and said, "Sister this is the young man that I was telling you about last night."

I gently held her hand, and the Nun placed the flowers on the end of her bed.

Suddenly I got an uncontroable impulse to smell the flowers.

I put my head over the flowers and I sniffed in, as my eyes focused on all the different colours.

For a brief moment my mind went blank.

I felt a swift moment of bliss, and that felt like I was dwelling at the centre of the universe for a micro second. I spent at least an half an hour with the lady.

The lady thanked me for my company.

I kissed her on the cheek and said God bless and waved to her as I left the ward.

As I made my way back to my ward, I felt a natural sense of wellness.

I suddenly realised that the helping of others is a true measure of ourselves, and by helping others we are truly helping our selves.

As I wheeled myself back to my ward, I thought with a childish enthusiasm. I am not going to meet the two thousand year old long haired happy hippy any time in the near future.

All my thoughts for the rest of that day were on going home.

I found it impossible to physically settle down.

It was one of the slowest days of my life.

I was in and out of the bed like a jumping jack rabbit.

As day became night I eventually began to steady my body and settle down.

My mind was still firing on all four cylinders.

The only way I knew how to combat this was to pray.

I grabbed my Beads from around Kidneys neck, and began to recite the Rosary.

After a few decades of the rosary my mind began to have deep thoughts and reflections on God.

Deep within me I sensed that the last rights and sacraments had put me back on the road to recovery.

I understood that miracles, can, will, and, do happen.

It felt like God had revealed how powerful he and I are.

I also accepted that my thoughts will shape and sharpen and change my future.

I accepted all my thoughts, feelings, and emotions, with openness, compassion, and love. Resistance to these thoughts seemed futile.

As my thoughts deepened I realised that all my life I had no one to love me on the inside, and life itself got in the way of all my dreams.

I realised that my reactions to other people's actions was the sole source of my disturbed mind.

I thank the heavens for my deep insights, and wisdom, and courage that was flowing through me as I prayed and gave thanks for life itself.

I know now that God makes us all remarkable human beings, but somewhere down the line with the burdens of life, we reverse the process, and make ourselves unremarkable human beings.

Our reactions or our non reaction to all things big and small is what truly makes us who we really are.

Suddenly my phone rang, and popped me out of my prayer and meditated induced state.

I answered, it was Mary she said, "How are things Tony."

I told her that I was fine, and if all went well I would be home tomorrow.

I told her I missed her and the children big time.

We chatted for at least twenty minutes and then we both hung up.

I snuggled into Kidney and I tried to drift off to sleep but it was near impossible.

I felt like a child waiting to go to Disney Land.

I called Israel over and asked him for a sleeping tablet.

He left and returned a couple of minutes later, and passed one to me. I popped it in my mouth and washed it down with some coca cola.

Within five minutes I was out for the count.

Suddenly the squeaky wheels of my gormay trolley woke me.

I finished my breakfast and got out of bed, and put my new clothes on. As I pulled my new jeans up I suddenly realised that my staples holding the wound together were still in me, they ran from my belly button and nearly all the way round my back.

I lay back down and I waited for my get out of jail free ticket.

Within an hour Mister Murphy arrived at my bed side.

He looked at me and said, "I suppose you want to go now Tony, any questions for me."

I asked about the removal of my staples.

He answered and said, "Tony will you ask your G.P. to remove them in five days."

I asked him what medication I was on.

He stared at me and in a forceful voice said, "Water!"

I thought to myself is it as easy as that.

He asked me how I was going to get home.

I told him that my friend John was calling to collect me soon. I thanked him for his services.

He wished me a happy future and then he left.

I packed my bag and I tried to leave, but I was stopped by the sister of the ward.

She asked me to wait till my friend arrived.

I told her that John was already at the front entrance waiting for me.

She said God bless and so did I.

Thank God she didn't walk with me because John was in my imagination.

Chapter Sixteen:
The Journey Back

My body was hanging for a cigarette, so I asked a young Dublin chap for one. He gave me two and I thanked him.

I went back in the main door and bought some coffee.

I made my way to my car in the long stay car park.

I threw my bag on the back seat and got in.

I lit my cigarette and sipped my coffee.

I reclined my seat and asked God to be with me, and protect me on the journey home.

As I sat there my mind put me back into the hospital bed, and made me relies I had being to the edge of life and I returned with the help of God and his son.

I rested for a half an hour. I then rang Shane and told him the good news.

I started the car and drove off into the heart of Dublin city.

Within ten minutes I was lost.

It took me two hours of painful driving to get on to the N.11.

I stopped at a filling station and rested for twenty minutes. I turned my phone off and drove on as pain crept back in again.

I pulled in to a lay by and rested up for another half an hour.

I realised I had stretched myself too far to soon.

I had no choice but to bear the pain and drive on.

It was getting dark and I was only passing Gorey Town.

So from there on I took the back roads, in hind sight it was probably the worst thing I did in a long time.

The roads were in an awful condition and every hump and bump, and pot hole exaggerated my pain.

Eventually after the toughest day of my life driving I reached Mary's house.

Mary was standing in the porch smoking a cigarette.
Mary came to the car and told me that I was in a lot of trouble.

In my naivety I asked her why and how.
Mary told me that the security guard noticed me leaving the hospital on my own and he reported it to my ward.
Mary said, "Tony they rang me and told me if you didn't arrive within the next hour that they would have to ring the police."

I stood along side Mary as she rang the ward.
She told them that I had arrived safe and sound.
Then she said, "I told you he is one of the best driver's I've ever seen." She then hung up.

By now I was as weak as a kitten and my legs were barely able to support my body.
Mary helped me to the camp bed and I lay down.
The house was in a strange eerie silence.

Mary had shipped the kids and Lana off to their dad for a couple of days.
Two days passed by and I was still incapable of getting out of bed under my own steam.
I felt like I needed a months rest after the ordeal that I had journeyed through.

On the third day the kids and Lana returned to the house. They crowded around my camp bed and Mary shouted, "Kids give Tony some space."
This gave me a sense that things were returning back to normal.
A couple of more days passed by and slowly I was regaining some strength and hope.

Suddenly it dawned on me, five days had passed and I still had my metal staples in me holding my wound together.

I told Mary that I was told to get the staples out in five days.

She asked me was I capable to drive.

I just smiled at her and said I think so.

Two hours later I was in Doctor Rows office lying on my back getting my staples extracted. Each one felt like a piece of knotted string being pulled from my body.

The extraction pain was beyond belief.

Mark left the office and returned ten minutes later and asked me how I was feeling.

I told him that the pain was fading by the minute.

He gave me a packet of pain killers and advised me not to drive my car. He wished me well, and off I hobbled back to my car.

I returned to my house and made myself as comfortable as possible.

Later that evening I phoned Mary and I am sorry I did.

Mary accused me of having an affair in Waterford, with one of my good friends. This annoyed and agitated my whole being for this was not true.

I told Mary what to do with herself and I hung up.

I didn't need this extra drama in my life right now.

For the next week I barred her incoming calls and I tried to get on with my life as best as I could.

I smoked some weed in the evenings, and I read a couple of books in the days.

I picked up the post one morning and the first one I opened was from Waterford Regional Hospital.

It was an appointment to see a Consultant Oncologist by the name of Dr Paula Calvert, for ten o clock the next morning. I was a bit worried and I wondered what she wanted me for.

The following morning I drove to the Hospital and went straight to the waiting room and checked in.

Five minutes later I was called into her office and as we shook hands, I felt a certain sense of calmness and peace radiating from her presence.

She asked me how I was coping. I told her that it's a hard mental and physical road, but at least I am still breathing.

She smiled at me and said, "Good man."

She then told me that she was referring me to a Consultant Nephrologists in the Kidney unit in Waterford regional hospital. I thanked her and then left and made my way home.

As I turned into my housing estate, lo and behold Mary was in my driveway sitting in her car.

We looked at one and other and smiled and entered my house.

I made some Star Bucks and sat down and chatted.

Mary apologised and so did I.

She told me that the children were missing me, and I told her that I missed them.

We finished our coffee and headed back to Wexford in Mary's car.

I spent all of December 04 recuperating in Mary's house. I did odd easy jobs around the house just to keep myself occupied.

Christmas was soon upon us, and I felt for me it was a time to give thanks to the baby Jesus.

We had a wonderful Christmas, and we even had Shane stay for the festive season.

In early January an appointment arrived from the Kidney specialist, and soon enough I found myself sitting in his waiting room.

I was called in and reached out and shook his hand, oddly enough his hand shake was very feeble and week.

He introduced himself, and the next thing out of his mouth was, "Mister Power you're not going to have a long life due to your medical condition."

I stood up and stared at him for a brief moment, as I controlled my anger and fear.

Without thought I said to him do you think you're God.

He remained silent.

Then I told him to never call me here again, as I left his office I called him a pompous ignoramus.

I went straight to the patient care office, and referred my story to a young lady. The poor girl was more shocked than me.

She handed me some paper and a pen, and asked me to write a letter to the man in question.

She left the office and returned ten minutes later with coffee for me.

My letter was finished by the time she returned.

Basically the letter said how dare you plant seeds of Death in people's minds. I also wrote you're sacked.

The last bit of the letter asked him to plant seeds of hope and confidence in people's minds.

As I left the office I wondered how in the name of God a highly educated man can be so stupid and insensitive to people.

I returned to Mary's house later on that evening.

When I entered Mary was jumping around the house in the best mood I had ever seen her in.

I asked her was she all right?

She told me that her uncle had passed away in San Diego, and left her and her sister a million dollar house.

From that day on Mary seemed to be suffering from anxiety. She wanted her share and she wanted it yesterday. She also refused to talk to her sister; they had fallen out with each other in a big way over the years. That left me to do the business end of things for her.

The house had to be sold for Mary to get her payment.

It took five months for the sale to go through and no money had come.

In the middle of June Mary's sister rang me and asked me to put Mary on the phone. She told me it was imperative that she speak to her.

I passed Mary the phone and within five seconds Mary was balling her eyes out. She threw the phone on the couch, and cried like a hungry baby waiting to be fed.

Eventually she calmed down enough to speak.

She told me that her Mother was on her last legs, and can-sir had spread through her body. I tried bravely to hold back the tears but it was impossible at the time.

I advised her to get her ass over to the States as fast as possible.

I told her that I would take care of the children.

Mary said, "No they are coming with me, and so are you and Shane."

Over the next couple of days Mary sedated herself with some valium. She also stopped taking her anti depressants, which she had being on since she had her first child ten years ago.

A couple of days passed by and Mary began to say and do strange things.

Mary asked me was I her long lost brother coming to save her.

She also said that her sister interfered with her when she was a child.

With the state that I observed her in I felt it appropriate to call the doctor. As luck would have it the doctor's surgery was literally two hundred meters up the road.

Ten minutes later the doctor arrived.

He spent at least ten minutes with Mary in the sitting room.

He came into the kitchen and said, "Tony Mary needs to go to hospital straight away." I asked him what the problem was.

He told me Mary was in the middle of a nervous break down.

The doctor asked me to bring her to Saint Sennens in North County Wexford.

I phoned the children's granny and told her what was after happening.

Fifteen minutes later granny arrived and spoke to the doctor.

We went into the sitting room and Mary was lying on my camp bed. She was dopey looking and silent.

The doctor had given her an injection.

Granny and I helped Mary up, and we put her in the car.

The doctor rang the hospital and told them we were on our way.

Granny stayed with the children.

I drove to the hospital and brought Mary in.

The girl at the desk asked Mary her name address and date of birth.

Then the girl said, "Welcome back Mary."

Mary aggressively snapped at the girl and called her a stupid cow.

Mary said, "How dare you say I was here before."

My poor brain was wiped out at this stage. I felt sad and sore, for my pain had crept back in to my wounds.

A man and a woman appeared at the desk, and the woman handed Mary two tablets and a glass of water.

Mary swallowed them, and walked off down a long corridor with the man and woman.

The girl at the front desk asked me to come back in the morning. I told her it's not a problem and I left the hospital.

I sat in my car and bawled my eyes out for a good ten minutes. I wiped my eyes, and I rang Granny and asked her were the children all right. She told me that she had them over in her house, and Lana was still in Mary's kitchen.

I said God bless and hung up.

I drove straight to Mary's house and collected Lana, and then I drove to my house in Waterford.

By now my mind and body was dilapidated.

I made a big joint and smoked it too fast, and I vomited up.

Ten minutes later I went to bed, and Lana lay on the floor beside my bed. I prayed like thunder.

From the bottom of my heart and soul I asked the god of my understanding for help and strength, to battle through the difficulty's that Mary and I were having. Suddenly I realised I was telling God what I needed, and I understood that he knows exactly what I need, and when I need it. I felt empowered by my conversation with the boss man.

I eventually drifted off to sleep.

The following morning Lana jumped up on the bed and woke me up.

I quickly dressed myself I made coffee and had a cigarette.

Lana and I got in the car, and I drove straight to the hospital in Wexford. I left Lana in the car and I went inside.

I asked to see Mary, and I was brought to her ward straight away.

164

Mary was still sleeping. I sat by her bed and gently held her hand as she woke up. She smiled at me and said, "Thanks Tony." She asked me about the children. I told her that they were with Granny. I could see the tension instantly disappear from her face.

I gently kissed her and asked her did she want to go for a walk. She nodded and said yes.

I called the nurse and asked her could we go into the gardens.

She answered and said, "No problem but be back before half past eleven, because Mary has an appointment with a team of specialists." I thanked her and we left the ward. We walked out into the blazing sun and,

We sat on the grass and hugged each other.

Suddenly I remembered Lana.

I told Mary that I had left my phone in the car, and I would be back in two minutes.

A couple of minutes later I returned with Lana on her lead.

As soon as Mary saw Lana her eyes lit up as if she just found a long lost friend.

Mary and Lana lay on the grass, and Mary hugged Lana to bits, and she cried for at least ten minutes.

I looked at them, and I sensed a sense of healing and happiness going on between them, and it felt like there was a tremendous field of energy and love enveloping them. Mary thanked me for bringing Lana to her.

Mary Lana and I walked to the car. I put Lana in and we went back in to the hospital ward.

Five minutes later a porter arrived at Mary's bed.

He brought us to a waiting room at the other end of the old red brick hospital.

We sat in the empty waiting room holding hands for a good twenty minutes, and then we were called in. I was ever so surprised that they called me in as well.

There were six people in the room, and we sat down at a big wooden oval shaped table.

One of the doctors asked Mary her name address, and date of birth.

Mary looked at him and said, "It's there in front of you."

A couple of people in the room giggled at Mary's statement. The man that asked the questions was not too pleased by Mary's reply.

Then he said, "Mary we're changing your tablets and we are keeping you here for a week of observation."

Mary stood up and said, "No way that's not going to happen."

I raised my hand and asked him what tablets he was prescribing for her.

In a snappy manner he said, "It's none of your business and I want you to leave the room now."

I stood up and with my dignity intact. I reached over the table and offered him my hand. He lowered his head and ignored me. I turned on my toes and said God bless, and walked out of the room.

I sat in the waiting room, and I could hear Mary blowing off steam, and putting him in his place.

The door opened and Mary walked out and said, "Tony please bring me home." I was appalled to think that this rude, thick, and, arrogant man was employed by the health board of Ireland for the people of Ireland. But I suppose every system has its flaws.

As I stood there people began to leave the room, and each one of them shook my hand and smiled at me.

Mister Thick was the last to leave. Again I offered him my hand as he hastily made his way past me. Again he declined as he sped his pace up and disappeared down a corridor.

Mary and I went straight to the reception area, and I asked to speak to the second in command. Five minutes later one of the ladies that was in the room appeared. She apologised for her colleague's behaviour. She sat us down and advised Mary to keep taking her tablets.

She wished us well and she left.

I went to Mary's ward and collected her bits and pieces, and we went straight to the car.

An hour later we arrived at Mary's house.

Mary got into bed and dosed for the rest of the day.

I phoned Granny and told her we were back home.

She told me that she would bring the children up later on that evening. She asked me how Mary was, all as I could say, was that she was in bed looking and feeling a lot better than yesterday.

I kept myself busy cleaning the house and looking after Mary.

Four o clock and my mobile rang. I answered and it was Mary's sister in California.

I told her about Mary's breakdown, she was very shocked and upset.

She told me that she was sending an international letter of undertaking for ten thousand euro to Mary's bank in Wexford town, and Mary would have to sign some paper work in order to release the money. We wished each other well and we hung up.

Five o clock came and granny arrived with the kids. They ran straight into their mother's bed room and jumped all over the bed. They hugged and kissed her. Granny pulled them off and told them to calm down. I made them both some tea, and we sat in Mary's room trying to make plans for the trip back to America.

Granny offered to mind the kids for a couple of days while we sorted out the finer details of our trip. Mary accepted, and an hour later the kids left with Granny.

Mary drifted off to sleep; Lana and I went to the Grotto in the garden. As hard as my life was I thanked Jesus Mary and Joseph for it.

I returned to the house and Mary was running around the house franticly prematurely looking for passports.

I asked her to stop and get back into bed. She sat on the bed and suddenly stood up again.

She reached under the mattress and lo and behold she pulled out the passports.

She handed them to me and I checked the expired dates on them.

They were all in date thank God.

Mary went back to sleep and I went to the sitting room and watched Coronation Street and East Enders.

Suddenly I wondered had Shane a passport. I phoned him and asked him. He asked me why.

I told him that Mary's mum was dying from can-sir, and we needed to get there as soon as possible.

Shane was fourteen at the time, and he said, "You'll have to ask my mammy." He put his mum on the phone, and I asked her could he come with us.

She asked me how long we were going for.

I told her of the situation, and I said I can't really answer.

She asked me when we were leaving.

I told her as soon as we can get a flight.

I asked her not to disappoint Shane.

She agreed and said, "You better look after him."

I told her that I would call tomorrow for Shane's passport and I hung up.

I was totally worn out from the day's events, and I felt a niggling pain in my latest scar.

I lay on the camp bed and I drifted off to sleep.

As usual Lana woke me for Pe. Pe.

I opened the back door and let her out.

I made some Star Bucks and then I woke Mary up.

I explained in detail what she had to do in order to get an advance on her money. I don't think she fully understood me.

It seemed like she was in a foggy state but stable, and at ease with herself.

We got ready and got in my car, and I drove to the bank in Wexford Town.

Mary tried to explain her case to the cashier but it came out all wrong. I took over and I explained Mary's situation in detail.

The cashier disappeared and returned five minutes later with a bunch of documents, and asked Mary to sign them.

The cashier told Mary that it would take five days to clear the money. I could sense that Mary was beginning to get upset.

I asked the cashier was it possible to see the manager, and with a slight resentment in her tone she said, "Yes."

We sat down and waited for at least ten minutes.

The manager approached us and led us to his office.

Mary tried to explain but she was getting mixed up with her words.

Suddenly she exploded into tears. I hugged her and I told her that everything is all right.

The manager quickly went through the paper work and said, "Mary I see you're waiting on a settlement of funds from America." Mary just nodded at him with tears in her eyes.

I gave him a small brief of what had happened, and told him what we would like to happen.

I also told him that time was the most important factor now.

He produced a form from a drawer in his desk, and he asked Mary to sign it. She signed it and passed it back to him.

He wrote out a cheque for ten thousand euro and handed it to Mary, and said, "I hope things work out." He told her to cash it outside.

Mary cashed the cheque, and we went straight to the nearest travel agency to book our flights to Los Angeles.

The woman there spent at least a half an hour searching the internet for flights.

The woman then said, "I'm so sorry, because it's so close to the fourth of July there is nothing available for Los Angeles until the tenth of July."

I asked her to search for flights to the nearest City to Los Angeles.

She asked us to come back in an hour.

We left and went to O'Brien's café and had some breakfast. As we sat there I noticed a strange bewildered look on Mary's face, her eyes were bigger than normal and protruding from her face.

I asked her was she feeling ok.

She said, "Tony I forgot to take my tablets and I feel like I am in a trance." I asked her where the tablets were.

She popped her hand bag up on the table and fumbled around in it for a couple of seconds.

She looked at me and said, "Tony they are in my bed room."

I left what was left of my breakfast and we walked back to the travel agency. Mary sat down and I went to the woman at the counter. The woman told me that the nearest airport was Toronto in Canada.

We got in the car and I drove straight to Mary's house.
Mary popped her tablets, and we had a Star Bucks coffee.
Mary and I got back in the car and I drove to Waterford.
I collected Shane's passport, and then I drove down town and parked the car.

Mary handed me three thousand euro and asked me to try and book the flights. I said are you not coming with me.
She answered me with one word, and that was "Shopping."
From that one word I knew that Mary's condition was stabilising and improving, and her eyes were back to where they should be.

Mary went on her merry way, and I went straight to the travel agency.
I was told the same thing that Toronto was the only alternative.
I tried another agency and again I was told the same thing.

I phoned Mary and five minutes later we met up in Mac Donald's. I told Mary that was our only option at the moment. She told me to go ahead and book it and said, "Tony we will probably get a flight from Toronto to L.A."

I had priced the fare and it was three thousand seven hundred. Mary gave me the extra seven hundred and she went one way, and I went and booked and paid for the flights. Our departure date was six pm on the first of July 05.

I phoned Shane and I gave him an update. He surprised me and said, "Dad I am fully packed and ready to go."
He asked me could he come with me now.

I asked him to ask his mum, and I would ask Mary.
I phoned Mary and told her we were leaving on the first of July from Dublin at six pm.
I asked Mary could Shane come down with us later on.
Love to have him was her answer.

I phoned Shane and the first thing out of his mouth was, "Can you collect me now dad."

I drove to Shane's house. I put his case in the car.
Shane hugged his mum and his sister and said, "Love ye."
I drove back down town and phoned Mary, and I asked her was she ready.

Mary answered, "Yes" and asked me to collect her at the main door of City square shopping centre.
I was surprised when I pulled up outside.
Mary had at least fifteen bags of shopping beside her.
Shane and I loaded the car. Mary got in and we drove to Passage East, and took the ferry way to Mary's house.
When we arrived Mary phoned Granny, and asked her could she bring the kids back.

I put a big mince stew on for dinner, and an hour later the kids returned home. We all finished our dinner, and Mary told the kids to start packing. Shane helped Adam pack his bag, and the two girls did their own thing.
Eventually the children were sent to bed. They were so excited and giddy it took them at least two hours to go to sleep.

Mary and I sat in the sitting room for a while tuning the finer details of our trip. She went to her bed room, and I lay down on my camp bed. My right side was acting up. I rolled a towel that I had borrowed? from the Mater Hospital up into a ball, and placed it under my right arm to stop my elbow from touching my side. I took two pain killers and I wrapped my beads around my wrist, and I began to ask my heavenly father to help me be strong for the journey that lay ahead. Suddenly I felt a deep sense of calmness and silence within my core.
It felt like my mind was on vacation from itself.
I was becoming my own best friend as; I was slowly being released from the realm of my can-sirus thoughts.
As my thoughts deepened I felt like I was the lead actor in my own film.

I asked my God to help me erase all my insecurities of my past.

The last thing that I remember that night was asking God to protect us all on our journey, and to keep me calm.

My pet alarm clock Lana woke me at six in the morning, and as usual I opened the front door and let her out to do her business.

I got dressed and got Lana's lead, and we headed down the road to the old Grotto by the railway tracks.

We sat down and my mind went blank. The more I tried to think the more my brain shut down. I felt a sense of emptiness and tranquillity. I never felt any thing like this in my life, and for a brief moment I felt at one with myself and the universe. Suddenly I realised that so far I had weathered the storm of can-sir, and I had transcended and transformed my way of thinking.

Suddenly I felt vibrations in the ground.

The early morning train was pounding down the track. I held onto Lana as the train roared by.

I felt a bit scared but excited like a child, as the old train thundered past us.

We walked back to the house and every body was up and dressed and fed.

Without asking I knew that Mary was ready for her second bout of shopping. I suppose like most ladies this was her therapy.

Mary left with the two girls and Lana.

I looked after Adam and Shane for the day.

We watched a couple of films and played in the garden.

Mary returned at six o clock, and as usual the car was full of shopping bags. I asked her where Lana was. She told me that she left her in the boarding kennels.

I had no dinner ready so I asked everybody what they wanted, and I made my way to the chipper.

I returned a half hour later, and we all sat down and munched into our food.

We eventually settled the kids down and sent them off to bed.

I re checked the passports and flight tickets.

I sat and asked Mary was she up for this trip.

She nodded at me and said, "Are you Tony."

I told Mary what ever it takes to get her and the kids there before her mum passes on, will be done.

Mary and I went to bed and tried to settle.

I was twisting and turning for a good twenty minutes.

I was disturbing Mary and she was getting a bit agitated.

I returned to my camp bed I cuddled into Kidney, and drifted into a prayer induced sleep.

The children woke us at six in the morning.

They were all wired to the Moon.

I got up and made pancakes for breakfast.

Mary stayed in bed and I fed the children.

I told the children to get dressed.

I brought them to the Grotto of Saint Patrick, and I asked them to say their prayers. We all returned to the house and began to pack the car. It wasn't long before twelve O Clock arrived.

Chapter Seventeen:

Finding Healing in the Madness

I drove straight to Dublin with only one pe.pe stop on the way.

We entered the airport, and I parked the car in the long stay car park. We went straight to MacDonald's in the airport, and we all filled up on junk food.

Eventually we all went through the departure gates without any problems.

Mary went straight to the duty free shops and, I took the children to the departure lounge.

An hour later we boarded the flight to Toronto Canada. We had a pleasant flight which took only four hours.

We arrived there at ten o clock that night. We cleared customs and collected our bags.

We got a mini bus into the centre of Toronto. We were dropped off at Mac Donald's

Mary and the kids stayed in MacDonald's.

I searched the centre of the city for a hotel for the night.

Everywhere I went I was told that the world convention of Alcoholics Anonymous was taken place that week end.

I tried one more hotel and they said, "Yes."

I quickly surveyed the rooms and to my horror the place was filthy and disgusting, and I got a sense of seediness from this place.

I returned to Mac Donald's and told Mary that it was impossible to find a place for the night. Mary started crying.

I asked her to stop and told her I would take care of everything.

I sipped my coffee and suggested to Mary that we would go back to the airport and, I would hire a big jeep.

Mary agreed and I went and hailed a mini bus.

We loaded up and were driven back to the airport.

We pushed our bags to the AVIS car hire centre with in the airport grounds.

I tried to hire a vehicle and everything was going well until the bloke behind the counter asked me for a credit card. Neither Mary nor I had one.

I offered him cash and he said, "Company policy no cash." Mary began to cry again.

We went outside and lit a couple of cigarettes.

At this stage the children were beginning to dose off on their bags. Come hell or high water I had to get the children a bed for the night.

I looked up at the sky and in my mind I said if your not on holiday O lord of the universe please help me get these children a bed and, in out of the cold.

I had no sooner said this and P.C. in Boulder City popped into my mind.

I told Mary that I was going to ring P.C.

Mary disagreed with me and said, "Tony it's the middle of the night in Nevada." I told Mary that I was thinking outside the box and I don't care who I wake up as long as I get the children out of the cold.

I went back to the AVIS office and asked the man could I use the phone. He passed it to me and I rang Paul's private number.

The phone rang out for a couple of minutes and suddenly P.C answered.

I told P.C. of our dilemma. He told me to put the receptionist on. I passed the phone back and five minutes later a two ton General Motors five point seven litre brand new jeep was at my side.

I looked at this enormous thing and I wondered would I be able to drive it. I told myself to cop on and in my mind I said, I can do all things through Christ who strengthens me.

I called Mary and the kids over and, we packed our bags in the back of this enormous land cruiser.

I turned the engine and the heaters on.

I went back to the counter and asked for a map.

I also asked the man was there any motels on the way to Niagara Falls. He told me that they were a lot, he said, "At least twenty."

I got back in the land cruiser and drove around the car park a couple of times just to familiarise myself with the controls of the cruiser

I drove out of the airport and onto the main road to Niagara Falls.

Twenty minutes later I felt a heavy thump at the front of the land cruiser.

Within two seconds a vile smell surrounded the land cruiser.

Suddenly Mary said, "Tony you hit a Skunk." I asked Mary should I stop. No way keep driving was her answer.

I drove on for a while and suddenly my eyes locked in to a sign on the side of the road that said vacancies.

I stopped the cruiser outside the main reception area.

Mary went in and booked the last room that was available.

We all went into our room and there were only two double beds there and they were six of us. I slept on the carpet that night and I didn't wake until seven the next morning.

Ten minutes later and everyone was up getting dressed.

I went to reception and got two coffees.

I called Mary outside the room and gave her the coffee.

I asked Mary did she want to go back to the airport and try book a flight to Los Angeles or San Francisco.

I was gob smacked when she told me that she wanted to drive the whole way across America.

I looked up at the heavens, and in my mind I asked god to take my fear away.

I looked at Mary and said lets go for it girl.

The children were thrilled to bits.

We packed the cruiser and I drove to Niagara Falls.

We spent a couple hours sight seeing, and then we left for the American border.

An hour later we drove up to the border in Buffalo New York.

Mary and her children had no problems passing customs.

Shane and I were held up and searched from head to toe.

An hour later and we were let go.

I drove hard for five hours. We reached Cleveland Ohio as the sun was going down.

Everybody was hungry so I pulled up at MacDonald's drive through on the outskirts of Cleveland.

Mary ordered the food. In my side mirror I could see two black men approaching the cruiser.

I locked the doors and I revved the engine.

I remember so well the look on one of the black mans face, and I think he remembered mine.

There was no hesitation in me.

If those two people had tried to rob us, I would have flattened them with the cruiser. Now my mind was made up and no way were we going to stay in Cleveland for the night.

An hour later we stopped in a small town called Cold Water. We had no problem getting rooms for the night.

The following morning we had our breakfast, loaded up and left.

I drove at a steady pace for eight hours.

By sunset we were on the east side of Chicago.

We booked into a small motel and had a meal, and we all went to bed.

The next morning I woke I felt a sharp consistent pain running from my belly button around my left side to the start of my back bone. I wondered was my Kidney failing.

I also wondered was I strong enough to finish this journey across America.

I took two paracetamol pain killers, and ten minutes later eighty percent of the pain had vanished.

We had our breakfast we packed and got back on the road again.

After a good six hours of constant driving we came to a city called Des Moines.

By now my pain was creeping back in and it was niggling away at my nerves.

I called Mary aside and told her of my pain.

We booked into a hotel and I went straight to bed.

Mary and the kids went for a meal, and a couple of hours later they returned.

I stayed in one room and Mary looked after the children in the other room.

Suddenly Mary woke me and said, "Tony its nine o clock."

I had being asleep for twelve hours.

I got out of bed and got dressed. My pain was still present but it didn't seem too bad.

We all had our breakfast. I filled a flask of coffee and we were on the road again.

I drove for about six hours and we stayed in Omaha Nebraska for the night.

The following morning I looked at my map, and I was surprised to see that we were halfway there already.

I drove on and reached the great plains of America.

Ten hours later I reached Denver Colorado. I was thrilled to bits I had driven past two time zones and gained a couple of hours of day light driving.

Mary asked me to stop in Denver.

I told Mary that I wanted to reach the Rocky Mountains before sunset.

With nervousness in her voice she agreed with me. I drove for an hour and the roads were twisty and steep.

The higher I drove the more nervous I became.

In the distance I could see lights and I made a decision to stop as soon as I reached them.

Ten minutes later I stopped in a small town at least three thousand feet up in the mountains.

We got a family room in a nice hotel for the night.

The following morning I was first to wake up.

I looked out the window, and I could see a snow capped mountain peak it looked like a Christmas pudding with icing on top. That sight made my day.

I woke Mary and the children up and pointed towards the mountains. They were as excited as me to see the snow capped mountain that looked like a Christmas pudding.

We had our breakfast and loaded up and I drove on.

It took a full ten hours of one hundred percent focused driving to complete the journey over the Rockies.

I stopped at a small motel at the bottom of the mountains.

We camped down for the night, and the following morning we were on the road again. I drove like a bat out of hell for ten hours and made it to Las Vegas at ten in the night. I drove down the main strip and asked the kids to roll down the windows. I popped a U2 c.d. into the player and I blasted out the song, the streets have no name.

The children and Mary were singing at the top end of their voices. There was a wonderful atmosphere in the cruiser that evening.

I drove to the Railroad pass hotel which was only two miles away from Boulder City, and we bunked down for the night.

The following morning we all woke at about seven o clock. We went down for breakfast.

During breakfast Mary rang Theresa and told her we were in Boulder City. Ten minutes later P.C. and Theresa arrived in the lobby.

Mary walked over to them and I stayed sitting down with the children.

Suddenly out of the blue Mary started to verbally abuse P.C.

I took the children outside and kept them busy.

Five minutes passed, P.C. walked out the main door and called me over to him. He reached into his pocket and took out his wallet, and asked me did I need money.

I shook his hand and said no thanks.

P.C. looked at me and said, "Tony please get her out of here as soon as possible." P.C. gave the four children a hundred dollars each. I stood there and I wondered what went wrong.

I thanked P.C for his help and support over the last nine months.

I walked P.C. to his car and helped him to get in.

I asked him what all the commotion was about.

He looked at me and said, "Family history Tony."

My earthly angel Theresa came to the car and hugged me and said, "Tony you have a hard journey ahead, be calm and patient and ring me any time, day or night if you need help."

I thanked them for their kindness and then they drove off.

I brought the children back into the hotel.

I went straight to Mary and asked her was she ready to go.

Chapter Eighteen:
Temper Tantrums

Mary snapped and said, "We are staying here for another night." I asked her what her problem was. She never answered me she just walked away and went to the room.

I asked the children did they want to go swimming in the pool they all said yes. I walked them to their room and they got ready for swimming.

We went straight to the swimming pool and they all jumped in and had some fun.

Fifteen minutes later Mary arrived at the pool and jumped in.

Straight away Mary got a hold of Shane and bent his fingers. Shane was hurt and upset.

I told Shane to get out of the pool, and he did.

Mary got out of the pool and started to abuse me.

I snapped and told her that she was out of order.

She called me all the names under the sun.

I left Mary and her kids by the pool.

Shane and I were fuming by Mary's actions.

We made our way to the cruiser.

I was angry and I decided I needed some time out.

I drove off towards Hoover Dam. I needed quiet time to cool down.

Three quarters of an hour later my cell phone rang.

I answered it was Theresa.

She told me to get back to the hotel right away.

I asked her why. She said that Mary had phoned the police and told them that I had stolen the keys and driven off. I asked Theresa to meet me there. I pulled into the car park and Theresa pulled in behind me.

Theresa told me to calm down; I took a few deep breaths and steadied myself.

We made our way to the room and entered.
There were three police officers in the room.
Straight away I was asked for the keys.
I handed them to a lady officer.

Theresa told the lady officer that the cruiser was rented through the Fisher Space Company and I had permission to drive it anywhere I wanted to. The lady officer asked Shane what happened in the pool.

Shane told the officer that he had accidentally bumped into Mary in the pool and Mary bent his fingers in retaliation.

The lady officer asked me what we were doing here.
I told her about Mary's mum's illness.
The police then cautioned Mary for false allegations, and then they left the hotel room.

Deep inside I was fuming, but I knew I was on a mission, and I knew come hell or high water I had to accomplish it.

I held Mary's two hands and asked her could we get on the road again she nodded at me as she cried, and said "Sorry Tony."

Deep inside me I felt I could feel her pain.
Theresa wished us well and passed me her private cell number and said, "Tony if you need me ring day or night."

I hugged and thanked Theresa, and then she left the room.
The children and I packed the cruiser and ten minutes later we were on the road again.

I drove as hard as I could, only stopping for food and pe.pe.

By seven that evening we reached a place called Bakersfield we booked a couple of rooms and bedded down for the night.

I switched on the television and to our horror it was a live broadcast for a missing two year old child.

We were all glued to the telly.

An hour later and the father with the child turned up at the police station. The children stayed close to us for the rest of the journey.

I lay down on the bed and within minutes I was out for the count.

Six o clock the following I woke to a sharp stabbing pain in my right side. I got out of bed and took three paracetamol. I popped into the shower and scrubbed up. Ten minutes later the pain started to slowly subside.

I woke Mary and the children and told them that this was the last leg of the journey. We all had pancakes and bacon for breakfast.

We loaded the cruiser and I drove off.

Every bump on the road increased my pain.

But I kept it to myself.

Five hours later we stopped for dinner at a stingy looking restaurant in the middle of nowhere.

We ordered our food and began to eat.

Halfway through our meal Mary's youngest girl said, "Mammy that man over there is staring and smiling at me."

I went to get up and sort this creep out but Mary pulled me back down into my chair.

Mary said, "Tony this is America and it's full of creeps and weirdoes just ignore him."

I uncomfortably finished my meal and we all left the stingy restaurant.

Even as we were leaving the creep still had his eyes on the child. I secretly wished I had a Hurley by my side that day.

As my pain was still niggling away at me, I drove rather slowly for the next four hours. Every bump on the road aggravated my pain.

Eventually I reached our destination San Jose at about seven o clock.

I stopped the cruiser at a nice hotel in the centre of the city.

As I got out of the cruiser I felt dizzy, and I presume I collapsed.

I came round in a couple of seconds.

Mary Shane and the hotel porter helped me up from the ground, and placed me on the seat in the cruiser.

Mary grabbed her phone from the dash board and began to ring the emergency services. I stopped her and told her that I was fine.

I sat in the cruiser for at least ten minutes and I tried to figure out what had just happened to me.

The porter loaded up his trolley and entered the hotel.

Mary and Shane helped me walk to the lift and brought me to our room.

I lay down on the bed and I thought of all the driving and concentration, and the pain and the drama in Boulder City.

I thanked God and myself for completing my mission of mercy.

Mary told me that they were going to see her mother after dinner.

I gave Mary the keys of the cruiser and told her that I needed to recuperate in bed.

Mary gathered the children and left for dinner.

I held my beads tightly in my hand and as usual I tucked into Kidney and I began to think deeply.

As I started to pray I felt a strange, but wonderful sense of achievement.

I understood now that this journey had worn me to the bone, and tested my stamina to the limits.

But yet deep inside me I felt that it was a wonderful therapeutic experience.

I looked at my life over the past year and I accepted that it was the toughest so far, and within that year I nearly met my maker. It was like an endurance test and I passed it.

The ultimate medal for this test was Life, and I was still breathing and trying to live the best I could.

I could see now that over the last year I done my utmost best to be positive. I felt like God and I had fashioned an escape route from death.

I realised that faith doesn't get to decide everything in life; we all have to decide some things in order to move on in life. In other words, [No guts no glory.]

As I looked back through time. It dawned on me that anticipation can do more damage than the event.

As I drifted off to sleep, my mind was at peace with itself.

Suddenly Mary woke me up. I asked what the time was.

Mary replied, "Tony its eleven o clock,"

I was confused because I could see light through the blinds on the window.

I thought it was eleven in the night but it was eleven the next morning. I slept for fifteen hours without waking.

I jumped straight into the shower and freshened up.

I asked Mary how things went last night.

Mary sat down and said, "Visiting time was up and they wouldn't let us in."

I pointed to the door and said lets go now.

Chapter Nineteen:
Half of My Mission Completed

We all made our way to the cruiser and I drove to the Home.

Mary went in and I stayed outside with the children.

She returned ten minutes later, and we all entered the home and made our way to Maria's, private room. When we entered her room it wasn't a very nice sight.

Maria was lying in her bed, and she looked like she was doped up to the eye balls, and close to the end.

Mary held one of her hands and I held the other.

Maria looked at her, and in a very low tone asked her to say the Rosary.

I began to say the Rosary and Mary and the kids joined in. Suddenly Mary began to ball her eyes out.

I continued praying and Mary continued crying.

I finished saying the Rosary and the room became quiet and calm.

I left Mary with Maria and I brought the children out side. I sat on a small wall and lit a cigarette and tried to reclaim my mental composure. The children were running wild in the gardens and I took no notice of them.

I felt so sad to have seen the woman that told me to pour the blood of Jesus Christ over my Kidneys nine months ago, withering away to nothing in her bed.

Twenty minutes passed and Mary stormed out the main door looking annoyed and angry.

I lit a cigarette and passed it to her.

Mary told me that a nurse came to change her mother's nappy and turn the pillow, and the nurse was very rough and rude.

In jest I said I hope you sorted her out.

Mary smiled at me and said, "Lets go for breakfast."

I rounded up the kids and we drove to a pancake house.

The kids ordered all sorts of toppings for their pancakes, chocolate, maple syrup, strawberries, and so on.

They all finished and they left a messy table behind them.

I drove back to the old folk's home and we all went in to Maria. All the kids kissed her and held her hands.

She called me to her bed and asked me to put a video tape on for the kids.

She pointed towards her locker and I got the message.

I popped the tape in the player and we all watched a black and white film with Maria and Charles Bronson as the main actors in it.

She drifted off to sleep and we quietly left her room.

We walked back to the cruiser and got in. Suddenly a big black Land Rover pulled up along side us.

Mary looked over my shoulder and said, "That's my sister Debbie."

Mary got out of the cruiser and straight away she started to abuse Debbie.

Both of them said some horrible things to each other that day.

I got out of the cruiser and asked them both to calm down. Mary turned towards me and said, "Shut up Tony, its none of your business."

I zipped my lip and got back in the cruiser as fast as I got out.

A couple of minutes later Mary got in the cruiser and tried to say sorry. I half heartily accepted her apology, and we drove to a Mexican restaurant for lunch.

We all filled our plates and sat down.

Five minutes later I asked Mary did she take her tablets.

Of course was her answer.

I held her hand under the table and Mary began to sob.

In her upset mood she told me that she would never forgive her sister for interfering with her when she was a young child. She said, "That bitch ruined my life Tony."

I asked Mary for the sake of her Mother would it be possible to put this issue on hold.

I doubted Mary in Ireland when she had her break down.
But now I didn't know what to think.
We finished our Mexican and drove back to the hotel.
The children played in the swimming pool for a couple of hours.

Out of the blue Mary said, "Tony I want to move to a different hotel."
Without asking why I told the children to pack their bags. Ten minutes later we checked out of the hotel.

Five minutes on the road and Mary pointed to a big hotel that said self catering.

I drove in to the complex, and Mary went in and booked a couple of rooms for a week. I drove to our apartment and we unloaded and settled in for the evening.

Mary asked me to go to the nearest store for cigarettes.
I left and drove out of the complex and drove to the nearest store. I bought two hundred Marlboro light and walked out.
As I was getting into the cruiser Mary's sister pulled up along side me.
Debbie said, "What in the name of god is up with her."
We sat in her Land Rover.
She told me that no way did she interfere with Mary when she was a child.
I said that it was none of my business and I couldn't interfere.
She asked me where we were staying and asked me could she visit. I told her it was up to herself to make that decision.
I told her we were staying in the Los Gatos hotel complex just a half mile up the road.
I wished her well and she drove off.

I returned with the cigarettes, and told Mary that I had met her sister, and she asked me could she come over.

Mary ignored me.

I was asked to mind the children for a couple of hours.

Because Mary wanted to spend a couple of hours with her mother on her own.

I kept the children busy picking oranges from the trees and making freshly squashed orange juice.

I also let them have a swim in the pool.

Time passed quickly.

Mary returned at half past three and to my amazement her sister Debbie was with her.

I asked how her mum was doing.

She told me that her mum said, she wasn't going to die while we were still in San Jose.

Mary asked me to tell the children to pack.

I asked her what's going on.

Debbie said, "Tony you're all staying in my house."

I was a bit shocked but I went with the flow of things anyway.

Mary and Debbie went to reception and got her deposit for the week back.

Shane Adam and I packed the cruiser.

We drove to Debby's house and unpacked our bags.

The children were very excited and they played with Debbie's two young daughters. An hour or so later her husband pulled up in the driveway at about six o clock. He was a tall heavily built man. He had recently being appointed as a judge in the San Jose district.

He walked into the house and the first and only thing he said to Debby was get them the f--k out of here right now or I am calling the cops to remove them. Debbie began to cry and apologised to us for her husbands behaviour.

I called the children in from the garden and told them that we had to go, and I asked them to pack their bags again. They did and ten minutes later we were on the road again.

I spent the next couple of hours looking for a decent hotel or motel.

Eventually I found a lovely place with a pool and sauna.

We booked in for three nights.

For the next three days we drove back and forwards to Mary's mum. I did my up most best to hold things together, and I tried to please every body.

One morning while at the nursing home, Debby arrived.
she got out of her land rover and approached Mary.
She asked Mary could she treat the kids tomorrow.
Mary looked at Debby and said, "Only if Tony goes with you." I agreed and then Debby went in to see her mother.
The following morning Mary rose early and told me that she was going to stay with her mother for the day.

As soon as she left I woke the children up and told them to get ready they did, and then I brought them to I Hop for pancakes for breakfast. They made a mess of the place and with embarrassment I found my self giving the server an extra large tip.

As we were leaving Debby rang and told me that she would collect us in an hour. We made our way back to the hotel and the children got packed and ready for their fun day out. Debby soon arrived and we all packed into her land rover. She drove for a good hour and then she stopped and parked in a massive car park.

We all made our way to the entrance of a fun park and Debby paid for the tickets.

As soon as we entered the children went wild and Debby and I had a hard time controlling and keeping up with them.

Over the course of the day all the children including my Shane vomited up due to the slides and rides.

All the same we all had a brilliant day, and I felt it eased the burdens of all our troubles.

Debby then drove us back to the hotel and we settled in for the evening.

Mary returned at ten o clock that night and I could see that she was very upset and tired. Before she went to bed she asked me to take the children shopping in the morning. I replied consider it done.

The following morning after a bad night of pain, and tossing and turning. I got up and tuck a couple of pain killers, and a half hour later I was feeling tired but the pain was slowly subsiding.

I woke Mary and the kids, they got dressed and we all had the hotel continental breakfast.

Mary then drove us to the centre of San Jose and dropped us their. We all had a brilliant day sight seeing and shopping and the day flue by.

At five o clock I rang Mary and asked her to collect us.

Mary arrived a half hour later, and we all got in and we went back to the hotel. We all sat and munched pop corn and watched a couple of films on television for the rest of the evening. Eventually we all went to bed.

On the fourth morning Mary surprised me and told me that we were leaving San Jose today. I asked her why.

Mary told me that her mum told her that she would not pass on while we were there.

I asked Mary where we were heading for. She looked at me with a bewildered look on her face and said, "Tony I don't know."

I asked the children the same question and they all said the same thing.

Chapter Twenty: Strange Happenings in San Francisco

Kevin, A friend of mine from back home in Waterford had an Irish bar in San Francisco. I suggested to every body that we go there. Everybody agreed and shortly after we were on the road to San Francisco. Before

We were halfway there I felt a tremendous pain in my chest, and I could feel and hear my heart raising its beat.

I pulled into a service station and told Mary.

Mary gave me two paracetamol tablets, and ten minutes later the pain eased off.

I asked Mary did she want to drive she answered, "No way Tony."

With one hundred percent concentration and effort I made my way to the outskirts of San Francisco.

As luck would have it, the first person I asked about Kevin's Irish bar, pointed me in the right direction.

Ten minutes later we pulled up outside Kevin's bar.

I scanned the area and it dawned on me that we were in the red light district of San Francisco.

I told everybody to stay in the cruiser and lock the doors.

I walked into the bar and ordered a glass of pure orange juice. When the girl gave me my glass of orange I asked her was Kevin around she said, "Yes he is in the kitchen, I will call him in a minute."

Suddenly Kevin walked out of the kitchen and in a loud half Irish and half American voice said who's looking for me.

I raised my hand from the end of the bar.
Kevin walked towards me and I moved my face out of view.
When he reached me I turned my head, and looked at him and held out my hand. When he recognised who I was, the look on his face was worth a million dollars.

Kevin and I were in the boy scouts as children, and as we got older we had a few pints together. We joined the reserve Irish Navy together and as life would have it, we pursued our own careers and went our own way in life.
It had being twenty years since I last saw Kevin.
I gave Kevin a short brief of the situation.
He seemed shocked and asked me what he could do to help us.

I then got Mary and the children and we sat in the eating area of the pub. I introduced them to Kevin.
He gave the children cold drinks and had a good chat with them. Kevin gave us his menus and said, "Lads dinner is on me."

Ten minutes later we were served our food.
Half way through the meal, and I was starting to feel unwell.
I began to feel dizzy as water poured from my face.
Again I could hear my heart thumping like the beat of a fast war drum. I was as red as a Wexford strawberry and I was really scared.

In my mind I asked My God to make sure I got the children and Mary back to Ireland.
Mary went to the cruiser and returned with my blood pressure tester.
I instantly wrapped it around my arm and took three readings, and the small watch like device worked out my average blood pressure.
The machine beeped and I looked at the final reading which was two

hundred and twenty seven over one hundred and sixty seven. I knew now that I was in the heart attack zone and I was really scared.

I showed Mary the results.
Mary said, "Tony I am ringing an ambulance right now."
I looked at Mary and said no ambulance.
I asked Kevin for a bulb of Garlic and a pint of water.
Kevin said, "Tony what do you want the Garlic for."
I told him that the garlic would reduce my blood pressure.

Kevin went to the kitchen and returned to the table, and passed me two bulbs of garlic and a pint of water.
Mary helped me peel them, and I ate them raw.
Fifteen minutes later I did the pressure test again.
When the machine gave me the average pressure Mary and Kevin were dumb struck.
The machine read one hundred and twenty five over ninety five.

At that very moment I suddenly began to feel and understand and accept the power of Mother Nature at her best.

This smelly small plant that Mother Nature provides was responsible for lowering my blood pressure, and possibly reversing the chance of a heart attack.
Out of the blue Kevin said, "Tony did you ever try medical marijuana."

I said yes Kevin you know how closed minded people are back in Ireland. He agreed with me and said, "Tony that's one of the reasons why I moved here years ago."
It was starting to get dark and the Irish bar was starting to fill up with all sorts of strange multi cultural people.

I told Kevin that we were leaving. He asked me to hang on till he packed our doggy bags.
He asked Mary had we a hotel for the night. Mary answered, "Not yet".
Kevin went to the bar and made a few phone calls and shortly returned to us.

Kevin handed me a piece of paper with directions to the hotel that he had booked for us over the phone.

The name of the hotel was the Cathedral, and it was in the centre of the City.

The girl behind the bar came over and packed the doggy bags. I stood up and she handed me the bag, and she hugged me tightly and said, "The carton at the bottom is for you, and get well soon man."

I really didn't know what she meant.

I sat down and Kevin said, "Tony there is a half ounce of Medical marijuana in the bottom of the bag."

I asked him how much I owed him.

He smiled at me and said, "Tony it's on the house."

Kevin walked us to our cruiser and we all got in and belted up.

I reached into my carry bag and I gave Kevin a small wooden box with a shamrock carved on top.

Kevin opened it and asked me what it was.

I told him that it was soil from the thirty two counties of Ireland. His face lit up as he thanked me.

We shuck hands and said our good byes, and I drove off in the direction of the hotel.

As soon as I drove off Mary

Questioned me about the girl that hugged me. I abruptly told Mary that she had no a thing to worry about.

A few minutes later and we were lost, and I was slightly panicking.

Suddenly Mary said, "Pull up pull up."!

I stopped and Mary got out and went to a taxi driver for directions. Mary got back in and said, "Tony follow that taxi."

The taxi driver drove off like a bat out of hell and I followed him, and struggled to keep up with him. This man was booting it through the streets of San Francisco.

The kids were thrilled to bits as we raced our way to the hotel.

The taxi driver pulled up at the Cathedral hotel, and I pulled in behind him.

I got out and gave the taxi driver twenty dollars, and told him that he was a brilliant driver. He said, "You're not to bad yourself." I thanked him again and then he spun the back wheels as he drove off.

Shane went in and got me a trolley and we loaded the bags on. We entered the hotel and while I kept the children busy, Mary went to the reception.

Minutes later Mary came to us and said, "The only rooms available are six six six and that's joined to six six seven."
The hairs stood up on the back of my neck.
We made our way up to our adjoining rooms and left our bags there. We left the hotel and went for a bite to eat; we came across a Chinese pastry cafe.

We gorged ourselves on all kinds of sweet rubbish.
The children were so happy to be out of the cruiser walking.

Mary held the two boys hands and I held the girls hands.
We all walked to the United Nations building in down town San Francisco.

I was surprised to see so many poor people hanging around the streets.
I felt nervous because there was so many poor people hanging out in door ways, and sitting on the ground, and I knew that before long we would be hassled for money.
I didn't feel safe there so I said come on lads we're out of here.

About twenty feet down the road Mary stopped and gave all the children five dollars each and asked them to pick a poor person and give them the money.
Lisa, Mary's youngest girl was the first to approach a poor woman sitting on a wall.

She went to hand her over the money and suddenly this woman spat on the child face, and told her to f--- Off.

I wanted to push this horrible person over the wall that she was sitting on.

Mary knew I wanted to engage, so she held my hand tightly and we all walked away.

Fifteen minutes later we were back in the hotel rooms. Mary put the children in room six six six and trough the connecting door we stayed in room six six seven. An hour later all the kids were fast asleep. Mary went to bed, and I decided to have a joint of medical weed. I rolled it up and went out onto the balcony and lit it. I slowly smoked it as I wasn't sure how strong it was.

It took me by surprise because five minutes later I had to sit down on the balcony. Ten minutes passed and it seemed like I hadn't a care in the world.

I sat there for at least an hour just staring at the lights of San Francisco.

My mind was blank and empty and it felt damn good.

I went back into the room and got my beads and Kidney. I went to bed and said my prayers until I fell fast asleep.

The following morning Mary woke me up at about seven o clock. I jumped straight in the shower and freshened up. I went to sit on the bed to put my socks on, and I noticed that my Rosary Beads were crushed and broke, and most of the plastic beads were split in half. I cannot explain what happened that night but it will stay in my brain for the rest of my life.

I called Mary and showed her the Beads. She looked at me and said, "You must have done that."

I said girl if I did that, I am sure I wouldn't have a tooth left in my mouth. She laughed out loud at me.

I quickly packed my bag and told the children to do the same. Ten minutes later we left the hotel.

I sat in the cruiser and asked Mary where to now?
Mary asked me to bring her back to her mum.

Chapter Twenty-One:
Back in San Jose

I made my way out of San Francisco and drove without stopping until I got to San Jose.

We booked into a nice motel only a mile away from Mary's mum. We just dropped our bags on the beds in the rooms.

We went and filled up on Mac Donald's.

I then dropped Mary at the nursing home.

I drove to the nearest park and I left the children run wild for a few hours.

Mary rang me and asked me to collect her.

When I pulled up at the home she was standing outside with an elderly well dressed man.

Mary called me over and introduced me to her uncle Stan on her mother's side.

Then she got the kids out of the cruiser and they all went into visit their granny.

Stan turned to me and said, "I hope you don't mind but Mary told me that you haven't being too well over the past year." I looked at him and said I don't mind.

Then he said, "Tony I am a retired professor of oncology do you mind if I give you some advice."

I said fire away as I thought to my self is this pure look or is it the work of God.

Stan told me to keep doing the same things that got me to this point.

He also told me to eat lots of nuts and berries, and then he said, "Tony, drink at least three litres of water every day between five in the evening and seven."

I asked him why between five and seven.

He told me that the body works like a clock and at certain times in the day our bodies will respond more efficiently. I thanked him for his advice.

We both walked into the home and made our way to Mary's mum. As I was walking I thought to my self the chances of Mary's mum's brother being a professor of oncology must be at least ten million to one or more. I felt now that this was a help and a sign

To keep going on no matter what happens.

When we reached the room Mary asked me to say the rosary.

I agreed and asked everybody to hold hands.

I said the whole Rosary as Mary's mum drifted off to sleep. We all quietly left the room. We said good bye to Stan and we drove to our temporary dwelling.

Mary brought the kids to the swimming pool, and I drove off to get pizza for dinner. I returned twenty minutes later and the kids munched the pizzas down. There wasn't even a crust left in the boxes.

We played card games for a while then Mary put the children to bed. Mary and I watched television for a couple of hours, and then I told her that I was going to have a joint.

I made it and walked outside to the gardens with Mary.

I lit my Joint and took a few pulls and suddenly Mary asked me for some. I passed her the joint and she had a few pulls. A couple of minutes later she asked me to bring her back inside. I held her hand and walked her back to our room. She lay down on the bed and fell asleep within five minutes. I went back out and finished the joint.

I sat there and wished we were all back home and safe in Ireland. I wondered how much stamina I had left in me. My thoughts deepened as the minutes passed by. I knew their and then that I would have to embrace all my fear and anxiety, and I had to try erase the battles in my mind. I had to embrace the negative as my own,

And hold on to the positive within me. That night I felt like I was in the darkness and the light at the same time. That night I sincerely asked God for a steady predictable life. I understood now that I was not going to experience a miracle unless I was willing to accept it into my heart. I preyed to God and asked for flexibility and receptiveness. I accepted the truths of my Can-sir, and for some strange reason this increased the level of my sanity. I was on my own out side in the cold, and I saw this as an opportunity to love and accept my self on a deeper level. I put my arms around my self and I actually hugged my self for the first time in my life, and it felt so good that I infused it into my daily life.

I made my way to the hotel room and went to bed.

The following morning the children woke me up. I had my shower and I felt calm and settled within myself.

Over breakfast I asked Mary what were her plans for the day.

Mary asked me to drop her off at the home on her own.

She told me that she had seen a play centre not far from here, and asked me to take the children there for the day.

We finished our breakfast and I drove Mary to her Mother.

I headed in the direction of the play centre but I got lost on the way. I rang Mary and told her I got lost, she told me to find my way to her sister's house, and she would direct me to the play centre. Instantly I said no way, but Mary reassured me that things were after settling down between them.

Ten minutes later with help from the children, we were in Debbie's driveway.

She came out to us and asked me what's up.

I told her that I was on my way to the play centre and I got lost.

Debbie suggested that we all go their together.

She went into her house and got her two girls and they got into my cruiser.

I drove to the Play centre and left the kids go wild for the day.

We sat and had coffee and began to chat.

In the course of our conversation Debbie said, "Tony do you really think I interfered with Mary."

I said I don't know what to think and it would be best for me to not have an opinion or take sides.

I told Debby all about Mary's break down and some of the strange things she said to me. Debbie said, "Tony I know what she's like and you're a good man to stick by her and the kids."

She told me that her husband had recently become a Judge in San Jose and he wasn't going to put up with any false accusations against his family.

I explained that when Mary had her break down, she said some things that I thought were out of context with reality.

The day passed fast and suddenly it was time to go.

I drove Debbie and the kids back to their house. Then I headed for the nursing home.

I arrived at the nursing home at half past five and I told the children to stay in the cruiser.

I went into the home, and Mary was sitting by her mother holding her hand, and sobbing quietly to herself. I sat down and I said a few prayers in my mind, for a safe and painless passage home for her mum.

By my observation of Mary's mum it was obvious that she had not much time left.

I asked Mary did her mother have the last rights.

She asked me to go to the nearest Catholic Church and fetch the priest.

On the way out of the home I asked the girl at reception for directions to the church. The girl said, "I will show you where it is."

She walked outside with me and pointed to a steeple about a mile away. I thanked her and I drove off towards the steeple.

Ten minutes later I arrived in the church car park.

I told the children to lock the doors of the cruiser.

I went to the house at the side of the church and rang the bell.

A small Chinese woman answered the door and asked me could she help me. I told her of the situation and immediately she picked up the phone and spoke to someone for a brief few moments. She put the phone down and asked me the name of the home, the name of the person and the number of the room.

I gave her the details and she told me that the priest would be there in a half hour or less.

I thanked her and we drove back to the nursing home.

This time I brought the children in with me.

They sat quietly as Mary was sobbing away to herself.

I told her that the priest was on his way.

I sat with her and told her that I think her sister and kids should be here.

Mary agreed and I went out of the room. I phoned Debbie and told her what was going on.

Ten minutes passed and Debbie and her kids arrived in the room. Shortly after the priest arrived, and introduced himself as Father Randy.

I found his name rather funny.

Father Randy took his bits and pieces out of a small black leather bag, and began to administer to Mary's mum the last rights.

When he was finished with Mary's mum he went to each person, and blessed us all in the room with holy water.

Then he wished us well and left the room.

Mary's mum pointed towards me. I put my ear close to her mouth, and in a broken low voice she asked me to say the Rosary. Mary held her mothers hand and Debbie held the other one. I placed the children around the bed and we made a complete circle of hands.

I said the Rosary and I was surprised that the children behaved themselves for so long.

When I was finished I brought the six children to my cruiser, and left Mary and Debbie with their mum.

An hour passed and Mary and Debby were at the cruiser.

Debbie got her two children and they drove off.

Mary turned to me and said, "My mum wants to see you Tony."

Shane was the oldest of the children so I asked him to hold the fort for a while. Mary and I went back into the home and as soon as we sat down Mary's mum asked her to leave the room. As soon as she left the room her mum held my hand and said in a crackly low voice, "Tony please bring them home to Ireland." I gently squeezed her hand and said consider it done. She thanked me from her heart for bringing her grand children to her.

Then she said, "Tony you've got a lot of light in your eyes please, don't let anybody steal it, and that includes my Mary." Her statement rocked my world.

I kissed her on the cheek and said thank you.

Mary came back in with two coffees and handed me one.

I sat in silence for a few moments as Mary comforted her mother.

Then out of the blue in a raspy low voice Mary's mum said, "Tony how is your Lung." At that moment I thought she was getting on to me for smoking.

Mary's mum asked us to leave and told us not to come back. Mary asked her why. She said, "Lads the time is coming and I don't want ye all to see me passing on."

I felt a wave of sadness as I burst into tears as did Mary.

We left the home for the last time.

We drove back to the hotel and tried to settle down for the night. I tried to cheer everybody up but my efforts were futile and unsuccessful.

A couple of hours passed and the children were all fast asleep. I made a joint and went outside with Mary, and we sat down and shared it. We both got very emotional, and we hugged each other as the tears slid from our faces.

Mary went back to the room and greedy me had another joint. I sat there and I wondered how in the name of god I was going to get us all homes safely.

I felt like I was in a shocking state of mind and I was only half way through this journey of mercy.

As I sat there I remembered Mary's mum telling me over the phone nine months ago, to pour the blood of Jesus Christ over my kidneys.

This broke me up inside because she had helped me in my hour of need, and there was nothing I could do for her in her hour of need.

Eventually I went back to my room and got into bed.

I got my beads, and I snuggled into Kidney, and I prayed myself to sleep.

The following day I was up and showered before dawn.

I went to the reception area and loaded a tray with all sorts of breakfasts.

I went back to the rooms and left the tray on the table for the children and Mary. I woke all the children up and told them to take their pick of the breakfasts.

Within five minutes the kids emptied the tray and asked for more. I made a second trip to reception and loaded up again. I left the tray on the table for the second time and this time it took them a little longer to empty the tray.

I then asked Mary what's our next move.

Instantly she said, "Tony will you bring us to Los Angeles." I said no bother girl just tell me when you're ready to go.

Chapter Twenty-Two:
Los Angeles

Everybody packed their bags and I loaded up the cruiser.

I drove off and made my way to the Pacific high way and drove down the coast for most of the day. I reached Los Angeles at six in the evening.

I drove to Santa Monica, and we booked into the original Hotel California. We put our bags in the room and went straight for a bite to eat. We came back to our hotel and settled down for the night.

We spent the next three days treating the kids.

We spent a day on Malibu Beach and another day on Laguna Beach.

On the third day in Los Angeles we drove to Venice beach, and I went into get some Star Bucks coffee. Mary stayed in the cruiser with the kids.

As I got close to the cruiser I could see Mary with the phone to her ear, and the tears were streaming down her face. I instantly knew that her mother had passed away.

I drove straight to the hotel and to tell you the truth I didn't know what to do or say.

I did my utmost best to comfort Mary for the rest of the evening.

I put the kids to bed and Mary and I sat their holding each other, and I tried to talk only of the good times.

Mary asked me for some Marijuana. I gave her a bud and she popped it in her mouth. Ten minutes later she was fast asleep.

For the next three days I brought the children to the beach while Mary and her sister over the phone arranged the cremation of their mother. Tension rose between the sisters as the days passed by.

Mary was insisting that her mother's ashes were coming to Ireland with us.

Her mother's last wish was for her ashes to be poured into the sea of the coast of Kilmore Quay in County Wexford. Mary asked Debbie to send her the key to her mother's apartment in Los Angelis. Debbie refused and a big row began.

She also told Mary that the ashes wouldn't be ready for two weeks. Mary then rang the crematorium and asked them about the ashes. They told her that they were ready to be collected.

By now the two sisters were tearing strips out of each other, and Mary's mood was starting to shift to a lower level.

I phoned Debbie and asked her about the ashes.

I was told in not a nice manner that it was none of my business, I hung up.

That night I sat down with Mary, and tried to convince her to go back to Ireland.

Mary was adamant that she wasn't going no where until her mother's ashes arrived.

We spent the next seven days wandering the streets of Los Angeles.

On the morning of the eighth day a courier arrived at our hotel room with the ashes in toe. I was over the moon, for I knew that we would be going home soon. I phoned Teresa and asked for her help.

Over the course of the day Teresa my earthly angel sorted out our air line tickets to Toronto Canada.

We were booked to leave in two days time.

I told Mary of the bookings, and she seemed to be in a state of mind where nothing really sunk in or mattered.

She asked me to take the children to Venice beach for the day, so she could get some time to process things in her head.

I asked the children to get ready for the beach, and ten minutes later we were all enjoying the sun, sea and sand.

At about five o clock the children and I returned to the hotel.

Mary was lying on the bed crying. I held her hands and tried to comfort her but she pushed me away and said, "Leave me alone." I left Mary in her room and I looked after the kids for the evening.

Eventually when the kids went to bed, Mary came out of the room and asked me for a Joint.

I made it and walked outside with her.

Mary smoked it all to her self in a couple of minutes, and she was stoned and wobbling all over the place.

I walked her back in and put her into her bed.

Five minutes later she was out for the count.

I Got Kidney and my beads and lay down on the couch, and began to thank the God of my understanding for his help on our journey. I preyed deep from my heart and sole and this made me realise that I had being to the edge of life and I returned. I sincerely asked God that night to lead us back home to Ireland safely.

The following morning when I woke I lay on the bed for a few minutes, and I felt a renewed sense of hope and determination to get us all home safely. I woke the children up. I gave them their breakfast.

I wandered off with them shopping for most of the day, and Mary again stayed in the hotel room.

When we got back I asked the children to start packing.

I asked Mary to come to dinner with us. She refused and said, "You bring them Tony."

I drove to a burger restaurant on Sunset Strip and all the kids really enjoyed the simple food.

I returned to the hotel and the children watched television for a while, and then I sent them to bed.

I asked Mary was she all right and I got no answer.

I sensed that she was fast asleep.

I found it hard to go to sleep. I tossed and turned for most of the night. I was over excited about the trip home.

Eventually it was time to get up and prepare for the journey home.

I popped into the shower and freshened up and dressed up.

I woke the kids and Mary and reminded them that our flight was leaving at eleven a.m.

When all the bags were sorted Shane Adam and I loaded up the cruiser. We had our last breakfast in the hotel and then we left for the airport.

I drove to the car hire centre and unloaded our bags onto two big trolleys.

I handed the keys into the Avis reception, and I was asked for my credit card. I told the man how and where the cruiser was hired. He tapped a few buttons on his computer and said, "Mister Power you are due a rebate of a thousand dollars."

I then phoned my earthly angel Theresa and told her about the thousand dollars and that we were on our way home. Theresa asked me to hold the line for a couple of minutes.

When she returned she told me that P.C. said to tell me that the money is a present from all in the factory.

I asked Theresa to thank everybody, and I said God Bless and hung up.

We all walked to the customs and security check area, and the kids and Mary went through first with me trailing behind.

Chapter Twenty-Three:
Busted

Suddenly I was stopped by a six foot tall police officer.

At that very moment I remembered that I still had a small bit of weed in my holdall. It didn't take him long to sniff it out.

He showed me the Marijuana and asked me was it mine.

I accepted responsibility and told him that it was for Medical purpose's. He began to book me.

I was bursting for a pe.pe. so I informed the officer.

The officer ignored my plea.

He told me to wait till his supervisor arrived.

I looked up at the officer and pulled my jumper up, and showed him my scars. I told him that it was a medical emergency. Then I told him that I only had four fifths of one kidney and if I didn't go soon I would be going into the danger zone.

Suddenly his supervisor appeared and he quickly informed him of the situation.

Instantly the supervisor walked me to the loo.

I unzipped and began to go, and suddenly the supervisor shined a torch on my little man. I was horrified.

I finished and he walked me back out of the toilets.

I stood facing him as he spoke to someone on his phone.

He turned towards me and said, "Mister Power it's an offence to be in the airport with Marijuana."

He sat down alongside me and I gave him a brief sketch of the last year.

He then said, "Mister Power you have had a rough year but I have to summons you and I don't want to but its procedure."

Then he told me not to worry about it because it was only a small bit.

He also reassured me that the District Attorney would drop it on medical grounds. He passed me the summons and he shook my hand firmly as he wished me well on my journey home to Ireland.

I walked through the departure gates and made my way to Mary and the children.

Mary and Shane burst out into uncontrollable laughing as I approached them. They both told me that I was an idiot, and I burst out laughing as well.

We were only waiting for an half an hour and then we all boarded the plane to Toronto Canada. It was a relaxing flight the children all slept for most of the flight.

We arrived there at half past three in the evening, and we had a stop over for two nights.

We cleared customs and I went straight to the taxi rank and ordered a mini bus to take us to a hotel.

Twenty minutes later and we were in our hotel bed rooms.

We left our bags there and went out for a bite to eat, and a good strong Star Bucks coffee.

I finished my food first, and I excused myself, and went outside to finish my coffee and smoke a cigarette.

I had no sooner lit my cigarette when a man approached me, and asked me for a light. I gave him my lighter and he lit his smoke. Suddenly I could smell marijuana.

I looked at the stranger and said is that a joint. He smiled at me and said, "Yes." I told the stranger what had happened to me in Los Angeles.

The stranger produced a small bag of marijuana from his pocket, and asked me did I want it for fifty dollars.

I gave him the money and he gave me the weed.

I made my way back into the restaurant and sat down. I waited till the children and Mary were finished their food.

We left the restaurant and walked around the City for a couple of hours. Eventually we walked the kids back to the hotel, and settled them in bed for the night. They all fell asleep within a half an hour.

I told Mary that I was going to the park across the road to smoke a joint. She said, "Tony you got busted in Los Angeles how come you have Marijuana."

I laughed and said jokingly he missed the big bit in Los Angeles.

Mary looked at me and said, "Tony you're mad."

Then I told her about the guy outside the restaurant.

I went to the park and had a smoke of the weed.

I returned to the hotel and ten minutes later it was lights out for me.

The following morning I woke early and I felt refreshed and recharged.

We spent all that day shopping and treating the kids.

When the children went to bed that night I went to the park again, and this time I had two joints one after the other. I was twisted beyond belief.

I made my way to the hotel room and lay down and I instantly drifted off to sleep.

Again as usual I was the first one up.

I took a cold shower and dressed.

I woke Mary and the children, and told them that our plane was leaving at one o clock.

We had our breakfast and the children finished packing their bags.

We went for one last walk in Toronto, and then we got a mini-bus to the airport.

As soon as I got the bags on to a trolley, I put what was left of my weed in my mouth and swallowed it.

We got on board the plane and as soon as I sat down the weed hit me big time. I felt as happy as a pig in s--- to be going home alive.

As the plane took off I began to say the Rosary and within a few minutes I was fast asleep.

Chapter Twenty-Four:
Back on Irish Soil

I was woken suddenly and the air hostess asked me to buckle up for landing. It seemed like I was asleep for a short while, but I slept for nearly the whole flight.

We arrived in Dublin at about six o clock. We cleared customs, and I rolled the bags to the car. With great difficulty we shoved all the bags in the car, and I made my way to the exit barrier.

I put my ticket in the machine to pay and the machine read three hundred and seventeen euro. I nearly had a heart attack.

I got out of the car and went to the parking attendant. I showed him the ticket he laughed and said, "Sir that's a mistake just give me seventeen euro and we will call it quits." I gave him fifty euro and told him to keep the change.

He thanked me and he lifted the barrier. I drove through and three hours later after a hard drive, we were home safe at Mary's house in Wexford.

We removed the bags from the car and dropped them in the sitting room. Mary told the children to dress for bed, and ten minutes later the house fell silent.

Mary went off to bed and I went to the grotto at the end of the garden. I sat on the bench, and I thanked every good source in the universe for getting us all home safely. I also under stud that the term, ask and thow shall receive was real for me. I got down on my knees and I cried from my heart and sole, in a grateful way for our safe jurney home. I felt a deep sense of accomplishment and peace.

I finished my prayers and I wiped my tears. I returned to the house.

Five minutes later I went to bed and snuggled into Kidney and drifted off to sleep.

The following morning when I woke I felt tired and weary, so I stayed in bed until eleven o clock.

Mary asked me to get up and collect Lana.

I drove to the kennels and collected her.

When Lana saw me she went bezerk she jumped all over me and licked and slobbered all over me. I put her in the car and drove back to Mary's house.

I pulled up at Mary's house and as soon as I opened the car door Lana flew out and hopped around the garden, and greeted each child one by one.

It seemed like Lana was happier then me to be home.

We all lounged around for the rest of the day.

The following morning I told Mary that I had to bring Shane home to his mum. Without any breakfast Shane and I drove to Waterford. I dropped Shane at his mum's house and I wished him well. I drove the short distance to my house.

I opened my door and picked up my mail.

The first letter I opened was an appointment for the end of august for the Mater Hospital. The second one I opened was an appointment for me to see the oncologist in Waterford regional hospital on Monday morning.

The rest were just basically junk mail. Later on that evening I returned to Mary's house. I was starting to feel rough and smelly so I decided to jump in the bath.

As I was sitting in the bath my mind flew back to Mary's mum. The words [how is your lung] seemed to be imprinted on my brain. I began to worry and wonder would the can-sir present itself again.

I settled my thoughts over the next few days, and soon Monday arrived and I found myself sitting in the oncologist's waiting room. Ten minutes later I was called in.

The oncologist introduced herself as Doctor Calvert.

She was a very pleasant and calm person. She looked and sounded so delightful, I temporarily forgot my troubles. She asked me how I was feeling, and had I any problems.

I told her that I had a constant niggling pain in my right side. She weighed me and measured my blood pressure.

She asked me when my next appointment in the Mater Hospital was. I told her at the end of the month. Doctor Calvert gave me a prescription for mild pain killers and said, "Mister Power I will see you again at the beginning of next month." I thanked her and left her office.

For the next three weeks I wandered between Waterford and Wexford. I did small easy jobs around my house, and Mary's house and garden, just to keep my thoughts away from what lay ahead for me.

The morning of my appointment in the Mater had arrived. I got out of bed at six in the morning and left Mary's house quietly.

I drove to Bray in Wicklow and parked the car in the train station. I got on the train and made my way to the Mater Hospital. Before I went in I had a coffee and a cigarette.

When I finished I went straight to the out patients department at the back of the hospital and booked in.

Ten minutes later a porter appeared and called my name out.

To my shock and my amazement the porter walked me to Saint Anthony's ward.

As soon as I entered Israel my South African friend approached me, and walked me to bed number one again. By now I was s------ my self in my mind.

I asked Israel why I had a bed.

He told me that there were three specific tests and they were keeping me in to monitor me.

Deep inside I began to panic. I had no clean clothes and very little money, and my cell phone was out of charge.

A half hour later a porter arrived and I popped into his chariot. He brought me to the scanning room and left me there. From a side door a nurse appeared and passed me a big jug of a watery like substance, and asked me to drink it slowly over the next hour.

The hour passed and the nurse returned and we walked into the scanning room.

I lay on the big tunnel like machine and the radiologists did their scans. I was moved to a different machine and more tests were completed. The last test was a brain scan. Ten minutes later

My porter returned me to my ward.

I lay fully dressed on the bed.
My head was full of fear of what they might find.
I wondered was the can-sir back with a vengeance.
I wondered how much time I had left on Earth.
I wondered was it all over for me?
I wondered was there anything that can be done for me now.

Israel could see that I was in an awful state. He asked me did I want something to quieten the mind. Five minutes passed and he gave me ten milligrams of valium.

He returned to my bed a half hour later and handed me a shopping bag. I opened the bag and I was very surprised to see a new pair of shorts a tee shirt and a pair of P.Jays, and a track suit bottoms.

I asked him where he got them. He told me he slipped out and bought them for me. I thanked him from the bottom of my heart.

I dosed in and out of sleep for the rest of that evening.
When it was late I asked for a sleeping tablet.
I was given two and that was lights out for me.
The following morning I was given a breakfast but I was in no mood to eat it.

215

At nine o clock I was told to get dressed and make my way to the consultation room at the back of the hospital.

I did what I was told and within fifteen minutes I was sitting in the waiting room.

After a wait of fifteen minutes my name was called, and I walked in to the room and sat down. The doctor sitting opposite me was in his mid twenties, he had glasses on, and he looked like a proper nerd.

He fumbled around with my files and scans for a couple of minutes.

He then looked at me and said, "Mister Power I am afraid its bad news." I asked him to be honest with me.

He told me that there were multiple soft tissue nodules within the right lung, and that they were highly suspicious that it was Can-sir. As soon as he said this, my world inside my head fell apart. He told me that in his opinion I had only six to twelve months left.

Chapter Twenty-Five:
Losing the Plot

I stood up and in a trance like state I shook his hand and left his office. I went back to Saint Anthony's ward and collected my few things. I then walked out the back entrance of the hospital.

As I crossed the road my mind was digging my grave.

Suddenly I heard a vicious screech of tires. I instantly turned and saw a bus a couple of feet away from me.

The bus driver pumped the brakes so hard that he slid of his seat and hit the inside of his window.

He steadied himself, and then he started to call me all the names under the sun.

I just ignored him and kept walking.

I made my way to the dart station and boarded for Bray, or at least I thought I did. My head was so mashed I got on the wrong train. When I realised I was on the wrong train I got off at the next stop and walked to the opposite track. It wasn't long before the next train pulled in and I boarded it.

Twenty minutes later I was sitting in my car in Bray, and the tears were like the Congo River in full flood. My whole body was shaking from pure shock and horror. I sat there and I tried to ground my thoughts but it seemed useless.

Fear was digging its nails into me.

Eventually I summoned up the courage to begin my journey home.

I prayed constantly as I drove, and I tried with great effort to keep my concentration up. Soon enough I was a couple of miles away from Mary's house.

All of a sudden for no reason that I can explain, I lost control of the car and crashed into a dyke, and hit a tree head on.

I got out of the car with no damage to myself.

I looked at the car and to my horror saw that it was written off.

I walked the country road to Mary's house.

Lana flew down the driveway and jumped all over me.

I pushed her away from me. I was in no mood for playing around.

Mary came to the front door and asked me what's wrong.

I walked straight to Mary's bed room and lay down on the bed. Mary followed me in and sat on the bed.

I told her about the not so smashing day that I had.

Mary made me a coffee and advised me to smoke a joint in the bird garden. Five minutes later I was in the bird garden.

I smoked a big fat joint, and it seamed like all my troubles were decreasing.

I went to bed that night and began to ask why me, and why again.

I wondered how long it would be before I meet Saint Peter at the pearly gates.

It felt like my life was quickly coming to a grand conclusion, and the small peace of serenity left in me was evaporating rapidly. Suddenly in my thoughts I realised a man without fear is a man without hope.

Slowly over the next few weeks I tried to gain back my mental composure. As I did I slowly began to realise that my only purpose was to live in the here and now.

Mary dealt with the car insurance company for me, and after three weeks I was sent a check for three thousand euro.

I went straight to the car dealer in wexford town and bought a small V.W. polo.

The following day I drove home to Waterford and sifted through my mail.

As the afternoon progressed I decided to take a trip to Mount Mellary.

I arrived at the Grotto in Mellary at about five o clock.
The place was empty except for a man in his mid seventies.

I said hello and he smiled at me.
I sat down and suddenly silent tears burst from my eyes.
The old man sat be side me and asked me was I all right.
Briefly I told the man about my journey over the last year.
When I was finished he looked at me and said, "I am a retired priest."

He told me that one morning while in Australia he decided to follow the sun from east to west.
He told me as he drove he was following the light.
I told him of my experience following the light in America.
He looked at me and said, "The chances of us meeting here are a billion to one." He also told me to continue following the light, and God would be merciful to me.
The old priest also told me to pray harder than before and believe stronger than before. I thanked him and I
Walked To the holy well and filed a few two litre bottles with holy water.

I returned to my car and tried to start it. The engine was turning over but it would not start. After ten minutes I decided to roll the car and jump start it.
The second I left out the clutch the car fired up.

All of a sudden a flush of goose-pimples stiffened on the back of my neck and shoulders. It felt like there was something not from this world surrounding me in my world.
I thanked the heavens and I drove home to Waterford.

As soon as I got in my front door I began to prepare some Esiac with the holy water from Mount Mellary.
I left it soak over night. The following morning I put the mixture in sterilised jam jars, and stored them in the fridge.

Suddenly there was a knock on my door I answered it.
My mum came in and I made her a cup of tea.

I told her that the can-sir had spread to my lung, she was devastated. She cried for a short while and then she stopped. She then told me that a black priest from South Africa gave her a recipe for lung infections a couple of months ago.

My mother asked me to come with her to the health food store. I sat in her car and waited while she went in.

Five minutes later she returned and handed me a jar of wild flower honey, and a bottle of Aloe Vera juice. Then she drove me to the off licence and asked me to get a small bottle of brandy.

Ten minutes later we were back at my house.

She poured the Aloe the brandy and the honey into an empty two litre bottle, and asked me to shake it for a couple of minutes. My mother told me to take one table spoon three times a day for the next month.

I sat down and I cuddled into my mother and I began to cry. I felt like a two year old child being comforted.

My mum eventually left, and as soon as she did I drank a full jam jar of Esiac in one swallow.

Ten minutes later I took a spoon full of my mother's potion.

I phoned Mary and told her that I was staying in my home for the night. Mary out of the blue snapped and said, "Well stay there for good then."

I hung up as fast as I rang.

I smoked a couple of joints and then I went to bed.

The following morning while I was in the bath my cell phone rang I dried my hands and answered it.

The girl on the other end introduced herself as Marian, Doctor Calvert's sectary and asked me could I come to the hospital after lunch. I said no problem and thanked her and hung up.

I pottered around in the garden for a few hours, and then at about one o clock I got washed and dressed for the hospital.

I made my way to a big corridor that was being used as a waiting room, and I joined Doctor Calvert's queue. I started to observe the people before me. Some had lost looking expressions on their faces. Some of the adults and children there hadn't a string of hair on their heads, and some were swollen from chemo therapy.

But yet we all had something in common Can-sir.

I was eventually taken into an examination room and asked to wait.

I took out my beads and I began to pray.

Suddenly a slim young well dressed lady entered the room. I stood up and as I looked at her I realised it was Doctor Calvert. She shook my hand and we sat down.

Every thing about her projected intelligence wisdom and dignity.

She said, "Tony I have studied your reports from the Mater hospital, and in my opinion it is not as serious as they made out." Her precious words helped quieten my racing mind. I felt now that there was a big possibility the young doctor in Dublin was totally wrong.

Doctor Calvert unknowingly by her kind approach had given me hope just by the tone of her voice alone.

She asked me what pain killers I was on. I told her I was not taking them, and I smoked a few joints instead.

She raised her head from her notes and said, "Tony we know your can-sir is genetic and environmental but please try your best to stop smoking."

I stayed quiet.

Doctor Calvert told me that she had made an appointment for Friday, for me to see a lung specialist in Saint Vincent's hospital in Dublin by the name of Mister Tolin. She passed me a brown windowed envelope, and asked me to give it to him on Friday.

I thanked her and said God bless and left her office.

Chapter Twenty-Six: More Scary Hospitals

Friday morning soon arrived I got up at six in the morning. I washed and dressed and had some toast and coffee. I got in the car and drove for three hours eventually I made it to Saint Vincent's hospital. I parked the car in the railway station directly opposite the hospital. I sat there for a short while and I asked God to be with me on the battles ahead of me. I also thanked him for the help in the past. I lit a cigarette and I concisely tried to relax my racing mind. I got out of the car and walked to the shopping centre near the hospital.

I bought a brown windowed envelope. I made my way to a bench in the grounds of the hospital and sat down. I wondered for a moment about opening the letter and reading it. I thought to my self its wrong, but I did it any way. It basically said that mister power has a tumour on the bottom of the right lung, and that there were spacious shadows on the left lung. For some strange reason I did not panic.

I felt like my higher power was with me and helping my spirit to relax. As I walked I realised now that even a bad day is a treasure and a pleasure. I slowly walked into the hospital and made my way to mister Tolins waiting area.

I checked in and the receptionists tuck my details. I was surprised that I was the only one there.

Five minutes passed and suddenly a door opened, and a tall well built middle aged semi grey haired man called my name.

I stood up and walked into his office as he introduced himself as Mister Tolin. He shook my hand with a firm and manly grip.

We both sat down and he asked me to squeeze his hands.
I reached over and I squeezed as hard as I could until he told me to stop. All he said was, "Very good."

Then he produced a small machine from under his desk, and asked me to blow into it as hard as possible.
I took a deep breath in true my nose and I blew for Ireland.

The machine beeped and Mister Tolin looked at it and said, "Tony you are healthy enough for surgery, and I am going to schedule it for the fourth of November."
I looked at him and said that's next week.
He wished me well and I left his office. I went back to the car and sat their, and I tried to gathered my roaming thoughts. I thought to my self I must have a peaceful mind if I want to have a positive healing. I made a decision to accept the trash in my head, and I truly accepted the path of can-sir as exactly where I am supposed to be.

I decided to drive to Mary's house.
Three hours of steady driving and I arrived at Mary's house.
I knocked on the door and Mary answered. She looked at me and said, "Why didn't you answer my calls."
I told her that I had a hectic few days with doctors and hospitals. I said sorry but she was still angry at me so I left and drove to the ferry in Passage. I boarded and soon I was on Waterford soil. Fifteen minutes later I was home.

I phoned my buddy Seamus and asked him to call up. A half hour later he arrived. We had a coffee and then he asked me did I want to go for a spin.

We got in the van and drove to Tramore.
He parked the van and handed me his bag of weed.
We made a joint each, and then Seamus took his two dogs out of the back of the van. He left them run wild on the beach, and we walked behind them smoking our joints.

An hour later and we drove home. He wished me well for next week, and then he drove off.

I settled down for the night and watched the usual crap on television. I stayed at home for the next three days preying, and trying to relax and take things easy. My son Shane wandered between his mother and me, and kept me company for those three days.

Soon enough Tuesday morning arrived I was packed and ready to go, and suddenly the door bell rang.

I answered the door I was surprised to see my oldest brother Jamie standing there. We had a coffee and a good chat about life. He gave me a book to read. I put it in my bag and put the bag in my car. I said good bye to Jamie and he drove off.

I made myself a strong Star Bucks and swigged it down. I got in my car and drove as I prayed the Rosary. I was soon at St. Vincent's Hospital. I parked the car in the railway station again.

I tuck a deep breath and focused my thoughts on positive healing. I smoked a cigarette as I walked to the main door of the hospital. I took a few deep breaths as I mentally prepared myself for what was ahead. I made my way to reception and checked in.

The lady asked me to take a seat. I sat for a good ten minutes and I prayed for a positive outcome. Suddenly a porter arrived and wheeled me to my ward.

I sat on the bed for a good ten minutes, and I tried to be calm and patient. Suddenly Mister Tolin arrived with two young men.
He asked me was I well? I just nodded and said fine.

Deep inside I wasn't fine I was scared more now than my previous surgeries.

Mister Tolin could read me like a book. He prescribed ten milligrams of diazepam, and asked the nurse to fetch it. Twenty minutes later and I was out for the count.

I woke during the middle of the night and I found it impossible to go back to sleep.

I snuggled into Kidney and I wrapped my Rosary beads around my hand. I lay their praying until the sun rose and shun its light though the ward windows. Suddenly I felt compelled to go outside for some fresh air.

I asked the sister could I go outside, and to my amazement she said, "Yes but be back in ten minutes."

I wandered down to the main door and sat on a bench outside. I tried to steady my roaming fears but it was near impossible.

A young girl in her twenties sat on the bench beside me and lit a cigarette. As soon as I smelled the smoke I asked her for one. She gave me two as she stood up and said, "Enjoy and good bye."

I sat their and smoked one after the other.

I eventually returned to my bed and lay down.

I began to browse through the book that my brother had given me. From what I browsed, the book immediately captured my interest.

Suddenly Mister Tolin appeared at my bedside. He looked at me and said, "I saw you outside, and please make that your last smoke ever."

I was given a blue paper gown and I was told to put it on. Mister Tolin said, "Tony I will see you when you come round after surgery."

I replied please God and his Blessed Mother.

The surgeon then disappeared from my bedside.

A half hour later and my bed was wheeled to the pre op room.

As they prepped me I wondered was I strong enough to survive my third major surgery. Shit I was scared because I was on my own. A nurse held my hand as they injected me with some greenish looking fluid, and that was it lights out for me. I didn't even get to count this time.

Five hours later I woke up and I was not in the same ward. I raised my hand and got the attention of a fair haired nurse. I asked her where I was. She smiled and said, "Tony you're in the high dependency unit."

She asked me how I was feeling.

I told her I felt like crap. I asked her to help me sit up in the bed. She called another nurse over and they took an arm each and propped me up in my bed.

Then the fair haired nurse gave me two pain killers and a glass of water.

From the corner of my eye I could see a rubber tube coming from the side of the bed sheets. I instantly pulled the sheets back, and I was delighted that the tube was not coming from my little man.

The tube was coming from my right side, and there was a small bit of blood in it. I got scared and I called the nurse, and I asked her what's going on. She smiled again and said, "That's only your drain bag and that's normal."

I asked her could she get me my book from the other ward, and five minutes later she returned with all my bits and pieces. I opened the book and began to read.

The name of the book was Tom Crenin an Antarctic explorer. The book was about the trials and tribulations of an Antarctic expedition. As I read on my mind started to visualise the scenes in the book.

A couple of hours later most of my pain had eased.

Suddenly I realised that the book had brought my mind to a very very cold place. It seemed like the coldness in my thoughts was acting like an anaesthetic, and as I read on I felt better in myself. I saw this as a mini Miracle. I said a few prayers and I thanked the heavens for being alive.

The following morning Mister Tolin arrived at my bed side, and immediately he checked out my drain bag.

"Very good," were his exact words. He called the nurse over and told her to remove the drain.

Ten minutes later I was free from all my connections and I felt great. I asked the nurse could I go for a walk.

She said, "No Mister Power we are transferring you back to your ward soon." Ten minutes later I was back in my ward.

I asked the fair haired nurse could I go for a walk.

She said, "Do you think you're strong enough."

I answered yes. Then she told me that she would have to ask Mister Tolin.

She disappeared from the ward and returned a half hour later and said, "Mister Tolin said yes but only a short one."

I made my way to the chapel within the hospital and as I entered streams of gratitude tears flowed down my face. I knelt down and thanked the God of my understanding for the third time. I sat there and I prayed the Rosary three times as a way of giving thanks for my life. I cried like a baby waiting for his bottle of milk. Eventually I wiped my eyes and

Left the chapel, and began to walk back to my ward.

I turned into a corridor and lo and behold my mother and her partner Jim were facing me. My mum was surprised to see me out of bed so soon.

I asked mum and her partner to walk me to the front door so I could get some fresh air. My mum held my hand as we walked to the Exit.

I sat outside with them, and I enjoyed the fresh early winter air, and their company for a good half an hour.

Then my mother hugged me and told me that she loved me to bits, even the awkward bits of me. Then she got up to leave, and to tell the truth I wanted to leave with her and Jim.

I returned to my bed and I began to read again.

I felt really comfortable within myself from my mothers visit. For a while I felt like nobody cared about me.

But now I felt the true love of a mother deep within my Heart and soul.

I kept reading as the days passed by.

A couple of days later my cell phone rang. I answered, it was Mary and she was in an apologetic mood. She asked me how I was. I told her fine.

She asked me to come to her place to recuperate.

I told her that as soon as I get out of hospital I was going to my home to relax and get well. Then she said, "Don't you love me any more."

I said you're hard women to love all the time.

She was not happy with my statement and she told me to go and f--- my self and hung up.

I switched my phone off and put it in my locker.

I was disturbed by the phone call so I picked my book up again and began to read again.

The reading made the days pass fast and all of a sudden Mister Tolin told me that I was being discharged the next day. He also told me in his entire career he had never come across a patient with a pair of lungs that were so big compared to their body size. He said, "Tony you have a pair of abnormal lungs they are as big as a horses, and they go all the way up under your shoulder blades." I thought to myself that God made me like this for this very reason.

That night it was impossible to sleep, my mind was all ready in Waterford, and my body was in Dublin.

I prayed for most of the night and as the sun rose I got all excited about surviving the third serious operation.

Now I had a sense that a force beyond my comprehension was involved in my life.

Mister Tolin arrived at nine o clock with too interns in toe. He asked me was I well; I looked at him and said thanks. I told him that I was feeling fine.

I was released at ten o clock and I went straight to my car and began to drive home. Suddenly my car began to start chugging and thick black smoke poured out of the exhaust. I kept driving and thank God the cops were not on the road that day, because they would have defiantly stopped me. I arrived at the bridge in Waterford at about two o clock.

Chapter Twenty-Seven: Back in My Home

Strange as it may seem as soon as I crossed the bridge the car stopped smoking. I made my way to my house and as I entered I switched my cell phone on. It beeped at least ten times. I looked at the phone, and it was Mary who sent me the messages. I didn't read them I just deleted them.

I phoned Shane and told him I was home. I asked him to call up to give me a hand setting up a bed in the sitting room, so I could lie back and watch the television in comfort.

Ten minutes later Shane arrived with his friend Keith.

Shane told me to sit down and take it easy.

Keith and Shane rearranged the furniture in the sitting room, and they put a small bed in the corner of the room.

Shane's mother collected them at about seven o clock that evening. I lit the fire and had a long soak in the bath. I popped myself and Kidney onto the small bed and began to watch television.

At about eleven o clock I got a compulsion to have a cigarette. I went to the back porch and lit one up.

I wasn't even finished when I felt like vomiting up.

I went back in and lay down, and I started to get extremely dizzy, so I sat up again. I barely made my way to the bath room and I vomited up. This went on for the rest of the night.

To be honest I really felt like there was something wrong and I was dying. I never felt so sick in my entire life.

Suddenly at six in the morning I realised that I had a nicotine patch on my upper arm, and the cigarette that I smoked set of some sort of a reaction within me.

I took the patch off and ten minutes later I began to feel a bit better. I then went back to bed, and I was so tired I went to sleep almost straight away.

At twelve o clock the following morning Shane rang the door bell and woke me up.

I got out of bed and let him in. I went straight back to bed. My body was as weak as a kitten.

This went on for several days until eventually I gained some strength back in me. As the days turned into weeks my mind and body were getting strong. My Good friend Seamus kept me busy hunting and fishing as often as he could.

One morning I answered the door and lo and behold it was Mary. She flung her arms around me and held me tightly. She whispered sorry in my ear, and cried her eyes out.

I made some Star Bucks and we sat down, and worked out some of our problems, and made up to each other. We both apologised for our stubbornness. Over the Christmas period Mary decided that she wanted to buy a house in America to rent out.

She asked me to go with her in March. I told her if all is well with me I had no problem.

The weeks passed by and suddenly March was upon us. I had no involvement with the organising of the trip.

Mary asked me would Shane be allowed go with us.

I asked Shane would he like to come with us and his answer was, "No way Dad." I think the last trip left him with bad memories.

Chapter Twenty-Eight: Hectic Lives

On the fourth of March we got a taxi to Shannon airport and at four o clock we boarded the plane for the States. We stopped over night in Atlantic City. Early The following morning we boarded a plane for Los Angeles. We arrived in L.A.X international airport at twelve in the morning. I collected our bags and put them in a large people carrier. The taxi driver asked Mary our destination. Mary replied, "Hotel California on Santa Monica Boulevard."

Twenty minutes later we checked in. Mary then took her children for a walk, and the porter and I hauled the bags to the room.

I gave the porter five dollars and he thanked me, and asked me was their any thing else he could do for me.

I looked at him and with a bit of hesitation in my voice, I asked him where I could get some medical marijuana.

To my amazement he said, "How much do you want."

I told him fifty bucks worth.

He disappeared and ten minutes later he returned and handed me the weed and said, "Enjoy sir."

I made one up and stood on the balcony and smoked it, as I stared at the blue shimmering Pacific Ocean.

My mind went blank and I seemed to be at peace with myself.

I lay down on a lie-lo and soaked up the California sun beams, and I thanked my God for all his help.

A half an hour later Mary and the kids returned.

Mary sat down beside me and instantly said, "Tony

Were you smoking weed?" I nodded my head, and she asked me where I got it. I told her from the porter.

Mary asked me to mind the children for a few minutes while she went to the store for cigarettes. Twenty minutes later she returned and handed me a bag.

I opened the bag and was amazed to see an ounce of California orange bud.

Mary looked at me and said, "Tony we are staying here for the week so enjoy your smoke."

Every day of that week Mary took the kids shopping. I spent the sunny days lying on the beach with an empty thoughtless mind.

I can deafeningly say that, that week was one of the best weeks I had since I was diagnosed with can-sir.

In the evenings when the children went to bed Mary and I sat out on the veranda, and we shared a few joints, and Mary drank some wine.

Our stay in the hotel California was coming to an end, so on the last night there I asked Mary where to next.

She said, "Tony I want to go to Santa Fay in New Mexico."

The following morning we all packed our bags and got a people carrier to the Trans Am central station in Los Angeles. We boarded a train for Albuquerque New Mexico, and fifteen hours later we arrived. We booked into a hotel, and we all were so tired we went to bed straight away.

The following morning Mary was the first up. She woke the children up and told them to pack again.

When they were finished, we went and had our breakfast in a small restaurant directly opposite our hotel.

A half hour later we were in a people carrier and on our way to Santa Fay.

We arrived there at eleven in the morning and checked into a motel. After we unpacked Mary asked me to mind the girls while she and Adam went property hunting. I agreed and five minutes later Mary left the motel.

I kept the girls busy for the day, we went sight seeing and shopping.

Mary returned at six o clock and told me that the price of property in Santa Fay was too dear.

I asked her what our next destination was.

I was surprised when she told me that she wanted to go back to Boulder City Nevada.

The following morning we made our way back to Albuquerque and boarded a flight for Los Vegas. When we arrived we took a people carrier to Boulder city.

We searched the town for a hotel or a motel but there was a convention on that week, and there wasn't a room available any where.

The cab driver suggested we go down to Lake Mead, "He said it's always quiet down there."

We arrived ten minutes later and thank God and his blessed Mother there was rooms available.

We checked in and dossed around the pool for the day.

The following morning Mary asked me to take care of the children, while she went to Los Vegas to do her driving test. She returned at seven o clock that evening in a foul mood, she had failed the test.

The following morning she left again and when she returned that evening she had passed her test.

I was worn out from minding the children, and the sweltering heat.

The following day Mary left again this time it was to buy a jeep.

The children and the heat were draining all my energy. I was feeling a lot of pain in my right side, and I was beginning to worry and wonder was my Kidney on its last legs.

Mary returned late that evening with a jeep, and she was in a good mood. She put the children to bed and we sat outside. I asked her to get us out of this sweltering dive of a motel.

The following morning we loaded up the jeep and drove to Boulder City. We found a couple of rooms in a nice motel in the centre of the town. I was pleased to be back in civilisation. We settled in and relaxed for the day by the swimming pool.

The following morning Mary told me that she was going house hunting again, and she asked me to mind the children. I agreed under stress and asked her to be back by lunch time. She said, "Yes" and drove off.

The children were getting out of control and my pain was niggling away at me.

Lunch time came and went and there was no sign of Mary returning.

Six o clock Mary returned and all hell broke out between us, basically it was about me minding the children for long periods of time.

By seven o clock I told Mary I was going home to Ireland.

I packed my bag and I walked to a motel across the road and checked in. I watched the television for the night.

The following morning I went for breakfast in Bobs breakfast bar. As soon as I walked in the door I saw P.C. sitting at the end of the bar munching a fruit salad breakfast. I was surprised to see him their. He called me over, and asked me to have breakfast with him.

He ordered a full breakfast for me, and we began to chat about my can-sir.

He told me that he could never forget the oncologist's words in Los Vegas.

He looked at me and said, "Tony you're not yourself." He asked me what the problem was.

I told him that I had a big blow up with Mary and I was planning to go home the next day.

P.C. stood up and said, "Tony I want you to stay and work for me as my personal assistant." He told me that he had a stroke six weeks before I arrived in Boulder City. I said yes but at the back of my mind I just wanted out of there. He had helped me true tuff times so I felt compelled to accept his offer.

P.C. told me to get my belongings and put them in his car. He handed me the keys and said, "Tony call me when you're ready." I went to my motel and packed my bags and checked out. I walked across the road and I put my bag in the boot of his car. I went back into the restaurant and told P.C. that I was ready to go.

Five minutes later I was driving P.C.s Lincoln Cadillac to the Fisher Space Company.

When I entered the factory, Teresa my guide and angel told me that P. C. had a stroke six weeks ago. She gave me some advice on how to handle and monitor P.C. She also asked me what happened between Mary and me. I gave her a brief account of the last week and told her that I was physically and mentally exhausted.

P.C. lived above the factory; he had it converted into a massive plush comfortable apartment with all mod cons.

Teresa brought me to my room and settled me in.

The Mexican man that had looked after P.C. for the last ten years without a holiday came to me, and thanked me for filling in for him.

Over the next couple of weeks I got to know most of the people in the factory, and I was doing well at my carer's job.

P.C. and I spent our time dining out in fancy restaurants and enjoying life to the max.

Suddenly over breakfast one morning P.C. said, "Tony Mary is saying bad things about you. P.C. told me that I could use his lawyers to sue Mary for defamation of character.

I looked at P.C. and said, there is no peace to be gained going down that road.

He looked at me and said, "Tony you're a wise young man." That morning P.C. told me to make my own path in life and don't follow anybody else's.

I loved listening to the wisdom of my ninety three year old friend.

The following morning I got up at six o clock. I walked to the car park to go for some star bucks. Right in front of me was a nearly new nine hundred c.c. Honda sports bike. I wondered what was going on.

I drove the Lincoln and got my star bucks and returned to the factory.

When I returned Teresa was sitting on the front step smoking a cigarette.

The first thing she said was, "Tony nice bike."

Suddenly it dawned on me that this was Mary's way of saying sorry. I was furious to think that Mary had tried to buy me over.

I kept the bike for five days, and in my spare time I rodded the beast on the desert roads of Nevada and Arizona. On the sixth day at six in the morning I drove the bike to Mary's hotel, and I left the keys with the receptionist. I walked back towards the factory and collected my star bucks along the way.

My head was all in a big mess again. I found it hard to be happy, but I did my best to deal with the break up of the relationship on a daily basis.

I tried to forget the break up as I got on with my duties as personal assistant to P.C.

Three weeks in and one morning a letter arrived for me. I opened it.

To my shock it was a letter from the court and a date to sit.

This letter was accusing me of threatening to shoot Mary, of stalking her and also of working without a permit. I felt sad for Mary for I knew at that stage she needed to forgive herself for the events of the past in her life.

Over lunch that day I showed P.C. the letter. He told me to calm down and let it pass.

Deep inside I felt like going home to Ireland, but on the other hand P.C. had helped me through one of the blackest moments of my life, and I felt I owed him.

P.C. could sense that I wasn't in a good place.

While sitting in his office he called Theresa to him, and mumbled some thing in her ear. Theresa returned to her chair and made a phone call, and suddenly switched it to P.C.

P.C spoke on the phone and he asked the guy on the phone to come to his office.

An hour or so passed and a big tall dark skinned man entered the office, they shook hands and then P.C. introduced me as his personal assistant.

P.C. asked me for the letter. I gave it to him and he passed it on to the tall man that was also called Paul.

The man read the letter and instantly picked up his cell phone, and walked out of the office. He returned five minutes later and said to P.C. "That's all sorted you'll have no bother any more."

Theresa made some coffee and P.C. Paul and I went into the conference room. We sat down and Paul the tall dark man took out something out of his inside pocket. He showed me a metal badge that said home land security, and he told me that he was in the secret service. I smiled jokingly, and then suddenly he pulled his coat to one side and it revelled his gun.

The tall man then said, "I have rang some body important in Boulder City and told them of the situation, and I told them that you're a gentle man and your ex is a tyrant."

The dark skinned man turned towards me and said in an affirming voice. "Tony you won't be bothered any more."

The man shook my hand and said, "Tony you are doing a good job here keep it up." He shook P.C.s hand and then he started to walk out of the conference room.

He turned his head and passed me his personal mobile number and said, "Ring me any time Tony day or night if you're in any bother while you're here." He said good bye and left the factory.

Later on that day P.C. handed me an envelope with my name on it, he told me it was my wages. I handed it back to him and told him that I wasn't here for the money.

I told him that it was my way of saying thanks for all his help in the past.

P.C. found it hard to accept that I wanted nothing from him.

By now P.C. had barred Mary from coming to the factory, and my job looking after P.C. was becoming really meaningful and spiritually fulfilling for P.C. and me.

As the days passed by I threw myself into my job and did the best I could.

One Friday morning a Pilipino doctor and his wife arrived at the factory, with this supposed cure for stroke victims.

I led them to P.Cs. office. They began to unpack their medical bag. P.C. asked them to go to his bed room and wait for him.

I asked Therese who these people were. She told me they were stroke specialists from Los Angeles.

I then helped P.C. to the lift and brought him to his bedroom. The so called specialists lay P.C. down on his bed, and hooked him up to a saline drip.

After five minutes on the drip they injected him in the arm with a yellowish substance.

P.C. drifted off to sleep and the husband and wife doctor team packed their bags. I drove them to the airport. As they left they said see you next week.

When I arrived back at the factory I was surprised to see P.C. up and flying all around the factory.

It took the best part of three days for him to slow down. The following Friday evening Theresa asked me to collect the doctors from the airport. I did and I dropped them off at the Boulder City hotel. The following morning the Doctors arrived at the factory and did the same procedure on P.C. as last week.

For some strange reason I did not like the Doctors.

I got a gut feeling that something wasn't right.

As soon as the doctors left, I got nosey and rooted in the waste bin beside P.Cs. bed.

I found the bag that this injection came in, and it had a complicated name on it.

I went straight to a computer and punched in the name on the label.

I was shocked when the computer described this substance as pure animal protein.

An hour later and P.C. was up and flying around his apartment in good form.

When Monday morning arrived I called Theresa aside and told her about my small bit of research.

Theresa looked at me and said, "Tony this treatment is costing seven thousand dollars a pop, and you're showing me the same thing is worth fifty dollars."

Theresa asked me not to tell anybody until she told P.Cs. oldest son Kerry.

Later on that day P.Cs. son approached me and asked me was it true. I looked at Kerry and said as true as I am standing here. Kerry thanked me for my powers of observation. He instantly phoned the so called doctors, and he told them not to come back or he would call the police. He gently broke the news to his father, and P.C. didn't seem in the least bit bothered.

Over the next six weeks one of my jobs was to stop all sorts of people from asking P.C. for money.

Every second day somebody from P.Cs. past would appear and try and tap him for money.

P.C was a generous man and he found it hard to say no to anybody. The harder I tried to stop him the more he went against me. I asked him why he was like this. He looked at me and said, "Tony you're too sensitive."

One morning a youngish lady and her six year old son walked into P.C. office.

P.C. introduced her as his new web site designer. Over the course of the morning it was obvious that she was another taker.

By two o clock that day the lady had P.C. wrapped around her fingers. This lady took an instant dislike towards me. It felt she sussed that I was on to her game plan.

Out of nowhere P.C. asked me to go to Debby in the accounting office.

Debby handed me an envelope and told me that there was a cheque for ten thousand dollars in it.

She also told me to keep an eye on things and the cheque.

Twenty minutes later P.C. I the lady and her son were in the Lincoln driving to Las Vegas to purchase a car for her.

We arrived at the car sales centre and I settled P.C. into his wheel chair. The lady took the wheel chair and asked me to look after her son for a while.

I brought the young lad out side and he played in a promotional bouncy castle for at least fifteen minutes.

I stopped the young lad from playing, and I went back into the show rooms with the young lad in toe.

As soon as the young lad reached his mother he told her that I had stopped him playing in the castle.

The woman looked at me and said, "Bring him out again."

I looked at the woman straight between the eyes, and, said love I am here for one reason and that reason is to look after my boss. I also told her that I wasn't her baby sitter.

I stood behind P.Cs. wheel chair for at least ten minutes while this woman was negotiating a deal with a sales man.

Suddenly a well dressed man approached me and asked me to control my son. He also asked me to keep the young lad away from the cars.

I burst out laughing and told him it wasn't my son.

The man said, "Well whose son is it."?

For pure messing I pointed towards P.C.

P.C and the man erupted with uncontrollable laughter.

The woman wasn't too pleased with our conversation.

The man asked me was I Irish. I said be gorra I am.

He asked me did I smoke. I said yes, he pointed to a side door and said, "Come on so." I asked P.C was he ok for a few minutes he raised his hand and pointed to the door without speaking. We walked out side and lit our smoke, and we began to chat. He introduced himself as the manager.

The first thing he said was, "What's really going on in there." I replied and said your guess is as good as mine.

He then said that's disgusting. I agreed with him.
He then spoke about his roots in Ireland.
He told me that his great grand father was from Kilkenny and he said, "I would like to go their some day and trace my roots."

We went back in to the show room and the woman was on the phone abusing somebody.
Eventually the deal was done and the woman had purchased a brand new Honda C.R.V. four by four.

I walked over to the manager and asked him how the car was paid for. He told me that it was on the never never, and that P.C. went guarantor for her. I then helped P.C. into the lady's new four by four and they drove off. I followed behind them.
An hour later we were back at the factory and every body there was gone home.

P.C. was tired so he went to bed and had a nap. The woman and her son made a quick exit in their new four by four. That was the last I saw of them.
The following morning Debby from the accounting department phoned me from her office, and asked me where the cheque was. I told her it was in the hold all on the back of the wheel chair. She asked me to bring it to her. Five minutes later I handed Debby the cheque.
She thanked me from the bottom of her heart, and said, "Tony we all love having you here, you've made our lives so much easier." I smiled at her and left her office. I felt great and I felt that I was in the right place.
A week passed by and suddenly one morning a tall elderly black man walked into P.C. office, and introduced himself as a faith healer.

After a few minutes this man began to hold his hands over P.C. head and began to pray. I could sense that this was a set up, but I waited for the right moment to intervene.

When the man finished praying he asked P.C. for thirty five thousand dollars to fund a spiritual hotel retreat in Las Vegas.

Theresa looked at me and pointed towards the door.

I instantly knew what she meant.

I stood up and said excuse me sir but P.C. needs some rest, would you please leave now.

The black man looked at me; he had a nasty look in his eyes. I walked him to the main door and that was the last I saw of him.

As the weeks passed by P.C. and I shared our stories of life and wisdom with each other. We were bonded by a sense of caring for each other.

One morning P.C. asked me would I go to jail with him. I was bamboozled by his statement until he explained why?

He told me that he was paying less tax than anybody in the factory and he felt it was unjust.

P.C said, "Tony I am not going to stop tax this week, and we will probably end up in jail by Monday morning." I wondered was he serious. I told Theresa of P.C. outrageous idea she informed P.Cs. oldest son Kerry, who was the director of the company.

Kerry spoke to his dad over the course of the day and persuaded him to back down.

The following morning over breakfast P.C. asked me to bring him to the credit union in Boulder City. We finished our breakfast and I drove him there.

He asked me to stay in the car while he went in.

Ten minutes later he returned with a bag of cash, and asked me to drive him back to the factory.

We went into his office, and he asked Theresa to put the names of all the employees on envelopes.

Theresa got to work straight away and handed me the envelopes. I went to pass them on to P.C. and he said, "No no Tony I want you to put one hundred dollars in each envelope for me."

I did what I was told and then P.C. stood up and said follow me.

P.C. got on his mini electric three wheeler, and we wandered around the factory and handed out the envelopes. Seventy two people that day were thrilled to bits so was I.

Later on that night P.C. told me that the measure of a man is what he does for others, not what he does for him self. I enjoyed his wisdom and knowledge and his courage to do the right thing regardless of the consequences. I learned a lot about life from P.C.

His wisdom was powerful. Each night while I was there we shared stories with each other.

A couple of weeks passed by and one night at three in the morning I was woken up by P.C. shouting out my name. I got out of my bed and went into the kitchen part of the apartment.

I was shocked to see P.C. lying on the ground twisted up in his walking frame, with a small trickle of blood coming from his nose. All as he kept repeating was, "Please help me Tony."

I quickly checked him for any broken bones.

I gently unfolded his legs and hauled him up on to his feet. I put his arm around my shoulder and hauled him to his bedroom.

On the way to his bedroom he stopped and said, "Tony I am sorry I s--- myself." I told him not to worry.

I brought him straight to his bathroom.

I helped him undress and popped him into his shower.

As he was showering, I brought his soiled clothes to a bin at the side of the factory and dumped them in.

I quickly returned to P.C. and helped him out of the shower, and I dressed him in clean P.Jays.

I told him that I was going to bring him to the hospital, he looked at me and said, "I am all right I just need some sleep." I helped him into his bed, and I sat down on the couch in his room. I stayed awake for the rest of the night and kept on eye on him.

Six o clock that morning Theresa was the first to arrive at the factory. I immediately informed her of the incident.

Ten minutes on and P.Cs. son Kerry arrived, and asked me why I didn't ring an ambulance.

I said because your dad wouldn't let me.

Kerry insisted that I bring him now.

I looked at Kerry and said, if you get him into his car I will bring him there.

After fifteen minutes Kerry got him to agree to go and get checked out.

Theresa and I drove him to the hospital.

As we wheeled him through the door of the E.R. room my eyes caught sight of a face that I had come across a couple of years ago.

It was the doctor that greeted me on my first adventure in that hospital.

He came over to P.C. and said, "Nice to have you here Mister Fisher." They spoke to each other as if they were old friends. As the nurses attended to P.C. the doctor looked at me and said, "Your face is familiar I met you before."

Suddenly it dawned on him and he said, "Holy God you're the man with the kidney problems." Yes I said and you're the man who pre diagnosed me, and that led to saving my life. The doctor asked me what I was doing back here. I told him that I was repaying a favour to P.C. for his kindness to me when I was under the weather.

Suddenly P.C. called the doctor and me to his bed.

P.C. asked me when was the last time I saw a doctor, and got a check up. I told him that I coutent remember. He chuckled at me and said, "Well we may as well get you checked out while we're here."

P.C. spoke to the doctor while Theresa and I went out side for a cigarette. When we returned the doctor told me to lie on the bed next to P.Cs. bed. I did and five minutes later I was having my bloods done by a small elderly gentle faced jolly woman.

Theresa sat between our beds and engaged us in some light conversation. Time passed by and both our results arrived at the same time.

The doctor went to P.Cs. bed first, and in a cheerful voice told P.C. that his results were good.

The doctor turned his head and by the way he was looking at me, I instantly knew that something was not right. He told me that my Creatine level was very high.

This scared me but I didn't let fear show.

The doctor disappeared and returned within five minutes. He handed me a tub of powder, and told me to mix a soup spoon full with water three times a day.

Then P.C. and I were released from the hospital.

We went straight to Bob's breakfast bar and munched into our food. Over breakfast P.C. thanked me from the bottom of his heart for my help over night.

As soon as we finished we drove back to the factory and P.C. went straight to bed.

Theresa could sense that I was out of sorts so she told me to go shopping for a few hours.

I drove to a place called Henderson on the outskirts of Las Vegas. I parked the car and I walked around for a couple of hours window shopping.

As I walked I felt sad lonely and isolated, and I missed my son and step daughter big time.

When I returned to the factory I told Theresa that I wasn't feeling the best. She looked across from her desk in the corner of the office and said, "Tony maybe its time to go home and take a break, and bring your son back with you." I agreed with her and I asked her to break the news to P.C.

When P.C. got out of bed Theresa called me to his office. I sat down and P.C. said, "Sorry Tony for being so much of burden on you, but you have been an inspiration to us all." He thanked me for being there for him and then he handed me an envelope and said, "Tony that's your wages for your work."

I said no I don't want it. He said, "Tony don't be stupid take it and have a holiday for yourself you've earned it."

I thanked him and I walked out of his office. I went straight to Kerry and handed him the envelope.

He asked me what was going on.

I told him that I was going home and that his dad had given me this.

Kerry opened the envelope and put the contents on the table. He counted the money as he passed me a small piece of note paper that was in the envelope.

The note simply read. "My dear and precious friend Tony please makes your own path in life and don't follow any one else's." Kerry put the money back in the envelope and said, "Tony there is three thousand dollars there, and as far as I am concerned you've earned a lot more than that." I thanked Kerry and he thanked me for looking after his father for the last couple of months.

Later that evening Theresa booked a flight for me to return to Ireland in two days time.

The next morning over breakfast, P.C. told me that he felt, and thought that he had not got long left.

I tried to console him by the fact that he was present in the room when I was given thirty days to live.

As we ate our food P.C. asked me could he come with me? I said no bother if you feel up to it. He smiled at me and said, "I am pulling your leg Tony."

After breakfast we returned to the factory and P.C. told me he needed to go for a nap.

I brought him to his bed room and he drifted off to sleep almost straight away.

As soon as he began to snore I left his room and went down to Therese. She told me to take the evening off and go shopping to keep my mind busy.

I got in P.Cs. car and drove to Henderson and began to shop. I bought some new clothes for myself and a few presents for loved ones back home in Ireland.

I returned to the factory just as Theresa was closing up.

P.C. was in his office. He asked me to bring him for dinner. I helped him to put a clean shirt on, and he told me to do the same.

When we got in the car, I asked him where to.

He said, "Tony to the Hilton in Vegas." A half hour later and we were both sitting waiting for dinner.

Over dinner P.C. told me that he felt close to the end.

He said, "When I go their Tony I will do my best to help you." I asked him to stop thinking and talking of death.

He smiled at me and said, "Tony death doesn't scare me any more as a matter of fact Tony I can't wait."

Then out of the blue he told me the when he was forty he came down with a bug that rose his temperature to the danger zone, and he was in an apartment on his own. He told me over dinner that was the closest he had come to death, and there was nobody there with him at the time except God.

He realised that night that the only one that could help him was God. He asked God for help and drifted off to sleep. When he woke his fever had disappeared. He realised that God had helped him.

He said. "Tony make the best of every breath that you take in, and start to love yourself more as you journey through life."

I thanked him for his wisdom and knowledge and his company.

We finished our posh meal, and then I drove P.C. back to his home over the factory.

I helped him into his bed and soon after he drifted off to sleep.

I went to my room and I packed my bag.

I tried to settle my mind but I was so excited about going home, it was impossible to drift off to sleep.

As I lay on my bed I wondered how Mary and the children were doing. I prayed for them, and I asked God to help Mary and the kids to find peace in their lives.

That night I knew that Mary and I were finished with one and other for good. It saddened my heart but some how deep inside I knew that if we stayed together, we would eventually wreck each others lives.

I sat in my bed room and I wrote Mary a long letter, and I did my best to use kind and gentle words. I set my alarm clock for six A.M. I must have drifted off to sleep because suddenly my alarm clock went off.

I got up and had a shower, and I tried to mentally prepare myself for the long journey home to Ireland.

I drove to Star Bucks and got some coffee, and then I walked across the car park and bought a big bunch of red roses. I then returned to the factory.

I wandered around the factory, and I gave most of the girls a rose each. One lady there cried and told me that when she woke today she felt terrible, and my rose brightened up her day. I said my goodbyes to all the kind people there. Time was ticking on and I felt myself getting anxious.

Suddenly P.C. appeared in his office with a sad look on his face. He tried to give me a thousand dollars but I profusely refused it, and I asked him to give it to the can-sir society in Boulder City. He eventually said, "Tony consider it done."

Theresa looked towards me and pointed to her wristwatch.

I instantly picked my bag up, and I made my way to the front door of the factory. I put my bag in the back of Theresa's red four by four, and I gave P.C. a big hug. I waved goodbye to P.C. and the others who gathered to see me off.

I felt so sad leaving P.C. for deep inside I knew I would never see him on earth again.

Theresa drove us to the local Star Bucks and asked me to get two coffees.

As I was leaving Star Bucks lo and behold Mary was standing in front of me, and by the look on her face I decided not to engage in any chit chat. I stood to one side and walked out the double doors.

Mary followed me and as I got in Theresa's four by four, she started to tell Theresa that I verbally abused her while in Star Bucks.

Suddenly Theresa snapped at Mary and told her that she was watching from her jeep.

She told her that my mouth didn't even open.

Theresa told Mary to cop on and grow up for herself, and then she quickly drove away.

On the way to the airport I asked Theresa to say the serenity prayer with me. I held her hand tightly and we said the prayer together.

As soon as we were finished I felt a sense of peace and freedom. At that moment I instantly knew that I was responsible for my own future, health, peace, and happiness.

Theresa dropped me at the main door to the airport and gave me a big hug and a kiss on the cheek, she told me to be happy no matter what. Then we parted.

I went straight to check in and plopped my bag on the moving belt. I gave my passport and ticket to the lady.

She handed me my boarding pass, as my bag disappeared from the moving belt.

I had an hour to departure so I wandered around the airport.

Suddenly my flight number was called out.

I made my way to the departure gate and joined the line. As the line got shorter I began to become excited at the thoughts that soon I would be back home in Mother Ireland.

I passed the air hostess my boarding pass she stamped it, and passed it back to me. I made my way to the door of the plain and handed the girl my boarding pass.

To my amazement she pointed me towards business class. As I walked to the front of the plane I wondered was this a mistake. I was directed to a plush chair and asked did I need any thing.

I asked the air hostess why I was in first class.

She told me that Mister Paul Fisher had rang the air port and upgraded me. I said really, she said "Really Mister Power."

I was thrilled to bits, and as I sat in my plush chair I mentally thanked P.C. and Theresa for their endless kindness to me.

As soon as the plane took off I drifted off to sleep. I woke an hour later and I was given a choice of dinners, T bone stake or Atlantic salmon and a glass of champagne. I totally enjoyed my meal and I drifted back of to sleep.

Suddenly the air hostess woke me up for landing in Atlantic City. I had a change over and I had to wait a couple of hours.

As I sat there I noticed a lot of soldiers coming and going, and I suddenly realised that these young kids were coming and going to Iraq.

Some how I could identify with them, because I had my own internal war going on in relation to Can-sir.

As I sat there I wondered how many would come back in black studded boxes. I felt sad for all of them. I said a few prayers for them as they passed me by.

The time passed by quickly, and I boarded the second plane to Dublin Ireland. As the plane took off my thoughts deepened. I realised that my breathing was very shallow. I instantly increased the rhythm of my breathing. Ten minutes passed, and from a simple thing like breathing deeply, made me feel fifty percent better than I was.

An hour into the flight and I was given a delicious spicy chicken meal and a side salad with a glass of Champagne. I munched my food down and quickly swigged off the glass of Champagne.

With a full tummy and a light headed feeling I drifted off to sleep. I woke an hour before landing, and I began to pray and give thanks to the God that I was starting to slowly understand.

I was positive that I was sharing my pain, and my fears and also my hope, and health with my God.

Through my prayers it seemed like I was being infused with the virtue of hope and acceptance.

I understood now that I am very un lucky, but yet I am the luckiest because I am still breathing.

I realised now that that every breath I take is a breath of pure life and joy.

Chapter Twenty-Nine: Back Where I Belong

The plane landed at four o clock in the evening. I cleared customs, and I got a taxi straight to Houston train station. I had to wait for the six o clock train to Waterford. I filled myself up with coffee and sat on a bench. I watched all the people passing by. I made a game of it. I wondered which people were well and which were not well.

Ten minutes before the train pulled away, I phoned Shane and told him to be at the train station by eight forty five.

I boarded the train, and within a few minutes I was drifting off to sleep again.

Suddenly I was disturbed by a loud roar, "Tickets please." I passed the conductor my ticket, and asked him were we far from Waterford. He punched a hole in my ticket and said, "About twenty minutes or so sir."

As the train rolled on, deep inside I began to get excited. I got so excited I began to cry.

As the train pulled in I wiped my tears with my sleeve.

I got my bag and made my way off the train.

As soon as I got off, my son and one of my friends Jason, was standing in front of me. I hugged Shane until he told me to stop.

I didn't realise how much I deeply missed him until I stopped hugging him.

Shane got my bag and put it in Jason's car.

Ten minutes later, I was at home in my small comfortable house at the top of the city.

Shane put the coffee on and Jason and I sat in the sitting room, and we chatted for a while about my health and my journey.

As Jason left he asked me would I be up for a spin to Mount Mellary soon. I said yes, but give it a couple of days so I can shake this jet lag off.
Shane and I sat in the sitting room and I fumbled through my bag.

I gave Shane some top class expensive clothes and runners. He immediately tried them on and thank God they fitted him.
Suddenly Shane's mum rang him, and told him that she would collect him in ten minutes.
I reached for my wallet and took out a thousand dollars, and handed it to Shane and told him it was for his birthday in a week's time.

The look on his face was well worth a thousand dollars.
I told him to treat himself to what ever he wanted.
Shane's mum arrived and beeped the horn outside.

As Shane was leaving I gave him a present of an expensive watch for Elaine, and I asked him to hug her for me. He said thanks dad as he got into his mothers car and they drove home.
I turned off the lights and I went straight to my bedroom.

I knelt down and said my prayers, and then I popped myself into bed. I grabbed my bunch of beads and I began to pray and give thanks for all that I have being through and for all that is ahead of me.

Suddenly the door bell rang I instantly looked at the clock. I was surprised to see that it was two in the after noon. I jumped out of bed and answered the door.
It was my good old friend Seamus.

I put the coffee on and we sat down and talked about the good old days when we were young.

As usual Seamus took out his bag of Cannabis and began to roll up. He offered me one but I said no thanks I am not feeling up to it.

We went into my small garden, and we relaxed in the early September Sun. Seamus made me laugh that day with his dry humour. I asked him why was he so happy all the time. He stared at me and simply said, "Tony I have only one life and I decided when my pop passed away, when I was seven to be happy all the time."

His phone beeped, he looked at the screen and said, "Tony I am on my way home the boss is calling."
As he was leaving he said "Battle on buddy no matter what."

I was feeling very tired and weak, and soppy and sad, so I lay down on my bed for a nap.
As I lay there I started to pray, as I was praying my mind drifted to a peaceful place. I nodded off to sleep and a couple of hours later my son Shane rang my phone.

I asked him was he ok, and was he coming up to the house. He told me that he was playing football with the lads, and he would call up tomorrow. I wished him well and I hung up.

Ten minutes later as I was doing a small bit of cleaning around the house, I suddenly remembered a dream that I had while I was sleeping.

In the dream I could see myself standing on a sloped concrete drive way, and the sun was belting down.
I was wearing a pure white tee shirt and a pair of short commando shorts, and a pair of white runners. This dream seemed so real to me.

I got on with my cleaning and when I finished I sat down and watched T.V. For what was left of the evening.

Eventually I went to bed, and the next morning as soon as I woke up I realised that I had the same dream again.
This same dream kept repeating itself for the next two weeks.

As I was making breakfast one morning my cell phone rang I looked at the number it was long. I rejected the call for fear that it might be Mary.

It rang again and I did the same thing.

Ten minutes later I got a text message and deep down I wanted to reject it, but my curiosity got the better of me.

The messages said will you answer your phone brother Tony; this is your buddy Niall in O.Z.

A couple of minutes passed and my phone went off I answered it. I was delighted to hear my mate's voice.

Instantly he said, "Tony my sister Skyped me and told me that you were sick."

In the same breath he said, "Tony get your arse over here as soon as you can." I texts back and said give me a couple of weeks, and we will see what happens. Over the next couple of weeks I began to seriously think of my friend's kind offer. One morning as I lay in bed I made my mind up to accept it. I sent him a text message and told him I was preparing for the long trip to Australia. Over the next week I sold my V.W. polo for two thousand euro and booked the flight.

I told Shane of my plans and from his heart he said, "Dad I love you and I want you to go, it might make you well and healthy again."

As he said this tears welled up in my eyeballs, and I struggled to keep them in, in Shane's presence.

Deep inside I wondered was my scar ridden body up for the long haul to the other side of the world.

If it wasn't it didn't matter because I made my mind up. I was going on a trip of a life time come hell or high water.

As the days passed by I began to get very excited and soon enough one morning I was on my way to Australia.

Chapter Thirty:
Unsettled

I took the train to Dublin City and a taxi to the airport.

I checked in and an hour later I boarded a plane to Frankford in Germany.

I stopped over for three hours and wandered around the airport. As I waited I stuffed my face with Mac Donald's and strong coffee. I felt like a child waiting for Father Christmas to come.

Eventually I boarded a massive plane bound for Singapore.

Eight boring hours later and I arrived there feeling tired but still excited beyond my expectations.

I stopped there for two hours and then I boarded another big plane to Melbourne. From there it was only a small short flight to my friend in Adelaide South Australia.

Customs gave me a bit of a going over, and they confiscated the excess cigarettes I had purchased in Singapore.

Eventually after twenty four hours of travelling I embraced my good friend.

He picked up my bags and we made our way to his jeep in the car park.

We were both over the moon to see one another because we hadn't seen one and other for ten years.

Niall and I got in the pick up, and Niall drove straight to the beach, and out of the ashtray he produced two joints of canabis. He said, "Tony puff away and wind you're self down."

I lit my smoke and puffed away.

Five minutes passed and suddenly I hadn't a care in the world.

We left the beach and drove to Niall's home.

By the time we got there, I was so tired I would have slept on a bed of rusty nails.

He made some coffee and we sat in the shade, and we spoke about the old times working together in Ireland.

He placed a bag of canabis on the table, and told me it was for me. I made one up and lit it.

Ten minutes passed and I said that I needed to get some sleep. Niall said, "Tony you go to bed and I will go and get some food for later."

He left and I went straight to bed. Instantly I drifted off to sleep.

For the next three days every time I opened my eyes a wave of tiredness and weariness covered my mind and body, and all I could do was go back to sleep.

When I eventually came round, Niall told me he was worried for me.

Over breakfast one morning he asked me was I up to doing some work. By now I felt a lot better in myself so I agreed. He told me that he had an easy job down by the harbour that was ready to start Monday morning.

Over the weekend we played a round of golf, we also went fishing and shopping.

Monday morning arrived and as soon as the Sun shone through the blinds, I got up and got ready for work.

I made myself a pot of coffee and went outside, and sat down on a bench in the shade.

As I sipped my coffee I suddenly realised that I was wearing similar clothes that I had dreamt about a few months ago, and I was feeling happy and healthy for the first time in years.

Being in Australia made me feel like I had not a care in the world.

Over the next ten weeks Niall and I had a ball of a time.

We did very little work and earned lots of money.

We always finished before twelve o clock, when the sun was at its peak.

As soon as we got home every day, I started smoking joint after joint and this always took my thoughts of dying to a different plane.

Not once while I was in Australia did my mind wander into the realm of can-sir.

I was ten weeks into the holiday and one morning I opened my e- mails and read through them.

The third one I read was from my earthly angel Theresa, and it read. "Dear Tony I am sorry to tell you that P.C. passed away three days ago, and he went peacefully in his sleep." I cried for a while.

I got on the phone and rang Theresa I asked her for the funeral arrangements.

That same day Niall drove me in to the centre of Adelaide, and we searched the travel agencies for a flight to Las Vegas.

With the urgency of the journey the best price we could get was nearly three thousand Australian dollars.

I had saved two and a half thousand dollars, and my friend paid the rest and said, "Tony when you are finished in the States, I made sure that you can change your ticket without charge to get back to Ireland."

Two days later I said goodbye to my kind friend and boarded a plane bound for the U.S.A.

As soon as the plane took off I wandered down to the empty seats at the back of the plane. I lay across two of them and I began to pray for P.C.s soul.

I drifted off to sleep, and twelve hours later the air hostess woke me and asked me to put my seat belt on for landing.

I was amazed that I had slept the whole way across the Pacific Ocean.

As soon as I got off the plane in Las Vegas a wave of depression disturbed my peaceful mind. I began to feel depressed and sad. I couldn't put my finger on what was making me feel this way.

I got a taxi to Boulder City, and on the way there I suddenly realised that my body was weak and my mind was up in a heap. I wondered had I done the right thing coming back here. The taxi drove me to the Boulder City hotel. I checked in and left my bags in the lobby. I walked to the factory and as soon as I walked in Theresa hugged me to bits as tears flowed from both our eyes. Theresa then said, "Tony you're just in time for Paul's service." She locked the main door of the factory and we drove to the church. It was a beautiful ceremony with lots of people there, including Mary. We totally ignored each other that day.

As soon as it was over Theresa drove a few of us to the after reception. I stayed there for at least an hour and then I began to walk back to my hotel. As I walked I cried and to tell the truth, I was very sad and miserable.

That night I went drinking and to tell the truth I didn't give a shit whether my kidney failed. I drank myself silly, and all as I remember is one of the factory workers helping me back to my hotel room.

The following morning I was still alive and I was very hung over and sick. I popped into the shower but it made no difference to the way I was feeling.

I went outside for a cigarette and suddenly Richie, a good friend of mine from the factory drove up along side the hotel and beeped the horn at me.

I walked over to him and he asked me what I was up to.

I told him that I was packing for my trip home to Ireland.

Richie asked me to stay for a couple of weeks with him.

I agreed and ten minutes later I was in Richie's plush trailer home on the outskirts of Boulder City.

For the next two weeks we had a fantastic time we drove all over Nevada in Richies open top jaguar, sight seeing. We also went to a few A.A. meetings and strangely enough these meetings helped me ground myself. Richie was a very wise man.

One morning over coffee he introduced me to his good friend an old Indian woman who was blind.

She asked me all about my journey that brought me here.

I blabbed on and told her my story. As she left that day she wished me well.

The following morning a car pulled up outside Richies home. The driver, who was Richie's brother and the old Indian ladies carer, came up onto the porch and sat with us and had coffee. We three men spoke for a while and the lady remained silent.

As they were preparing to leave the woman stood up and put her hand in her jacket pocket and pulled out a silver rope chain, and as she handed it to me she said, "Jesus deserves better than the string he is hanging from."

I looked at Riche and his brother, and wondered who told the lady about the cross with the string around my neck.

Straight away I asked the lady how she knew.

Young man she said, "I felt it." Richie his brother and I were speechless for a few moments.

The woman held my hand and said, "Tony the spirit surrounds you, and I can feel its presence as we speak." The hairs on the back of my neck and upper arms instantly stood up, as a shiver ran from my head to my toes. The Indian lady kissed me on the cheek, and then Richie's brother brought her back to the car and they drove away.

I put my cross on my new chain, and at that moment I felt a great spirit of hope and confidence over whelming me.

It felt like the weight of can-sir had being lifted from my mind.

Before I got can-sir I felt like I owed some sort of an apology to the world, and everybody in it just for my existence on Earth.

As soon as I put my new chain around my neck, I instantly got a heightened sense of my own self worth.

The couple of weeks flew by, and it was time to leave Boulder City again. Richie kindly sorted out my airline ticket. The following morning I made a quick visit to the factory, and I said my good byes to all my friends their.

Then Richie drove me to the airport and we parted in good spirits.

An hour later I boarded a plane for Atlantic City. I found it hard to mentally settle my self. I tried to sleep but it was imposable. After five hours flying the plain landed. I played slot machines for a while. I tried to pass the time because I had a stop over for four hours. Eventually the flight number was called. I made my way to the departure area and boarded for Dublin. I tried to settle again but it was impossible. I felt tired lonely and sad. I took my beads out and I prayed the whole way home. The plane landed in Dublin at about four o clock. I cleared customs and made my way to the taxi rank. I popped my bag in the boot, and we headed for the railway station. It took us nearly an hour to get to the railway station. I nearly missed the train.

I bought my ticket and I had to run the platform to board the six o clock train for Waterford. I tried to settle on the train but again my mind was racing, and a small bit of pain was niggling at my right side just above my hip.

Three hours later I arrived home to my nice little house at the top of the town. I went straight to bed and grabbed my beads. I prayed until I crashed out for the night. The following morning I phoned Shane and told him that I was at home. He was at my door within ten minutes. I hugged him to bits, and I made us some tea and toast. Over breakfast Shane looked at me and said I missed you dad. I instantly roared my eyes out, and I left the kitchen and tried to pull myself together.

Shane's mum collected him ten minutes later.

I had a long soak in the bath and I felt ten times better than when I woke up.

As one day rolled into another, as sure as God one month rolled into another. I spent a lot of time in the country side over the next six months with my friend Seamus.

We got up to all sorts of things like ferreting for rabbits, fishing for trout, hunting foxes and coursing the odd Hare.

There was also no shortage of cannabis.

At this time in my life I felt like God was giving me a holiday from my can-sir and from myself.

Everything was going smooth and easy in my life until suddenly one morning a dodgy brown letter arrived in my letter box. I panicked for a brief moment before I opened it, all sorts of morbid junk flowed through my head.

As soon as I opened the letter my heart skipped a beat.

Chapter Thirty-One:
More Can-Sir

It was a letter from the regional hospital for an appointment for a full set of tests in two weeks' time.

Over the next two weeks my up beat good humour began to waver. I gave it my best shot to be happy, but as soon as I thought of my up coming appointment my mood quickly shifted downwards.

Suddenly the waiting was over. I drove to the hospital and checked in to the can-sir day unit.

All my tests were completed within a couple of hours, and I was sent home only to wait another two weeks for the results.

After a week and a half of internal turmoil my cell phone rang at ten in the morning. I looked at the number and to my horror it was the hospital.

I spoke to a lady called Marian. She asked me would it be possible to be there at twelve o clock in the morning, and she also advised me to bring somebody with me.

As I left the phone down I felt like an earthquake had erupted in my mind. By the urgency of the appointment deep in side I knew that there was bad news to be swallowed down.

Later on that evening I bought myself a small bag of cannabis, and I drove to an old friend by the name of Annabel. I sat in her kitchen and smoked one joint after another. Eventually I told her about my appointment in the morning. She suggested that she come with me in the morning. I agreed and thanked her from all of my heart.

As I went to leave Annabel's, she looked at me and said, "Tony you're in no state to drive, please stay here for the night." I agreed with her and thanked her for her kindness.

Annabel made some coffee, and I made a few more joints, and I puffed them down like the big bad wolf.

Strangely enough I was not engulfed by depression or desperation, but inside tears gently and silently flowed.

Annabel showed me to my room and said, "Good night."

As soon as she closed the door I dropped to my knees. I began to ask my old friend God for the sanity to accept whatever outcome was ahead of me.

I had no Rosary beads that night so I prayed on my fingers as I drifted off to sleep.

The next morning I was up at eight I had a long cold shower.

Annabel rose shortly after me and shouted, "Tony breakfast on the grill."

We ate our breakfast and sat and talked for a while.

Time was moving on and we got in the car. Ten minutes later Annabel and I were sitting in an empty waiting room. Five minutes passed and suddenly Doctor Calvert walked into the waiting room. She shook both our hands and asked us to follow her.

We followed her to her consultation room and sat down.

Doctor Calvert, I sensed had a strange look on her face.

I was hoping for good news, but I knew by being asked to bring a friend that the news was not going to be good news.

Doctor Calvert told me straight up that I had four tumours two on each lung, and surgery was not an option.

My brain froze solid and from that moment on I felt muted. I struggled to hold back the tears.

Annabel and Doctor Calvert kept speaking.

I could hear nothing. I could only see their lips moving. My brain was like a sponge full of water and it could not absorb no more.

Doctor Calvert stood up and that was my cue to leave her office.

Annabel and I walked to the main entrance and lit a couple of cigarettes. I was in extreme shock from my head to my toes. Annabel went and got me some coffee.

I slugged the coffee down and smoked at least five cigarettes.

I eventually steadied myself enough to drive back to Annabel's house. As soon as I stepped into Annabel's house, she poured me a large glass of vodka. I swigged it down and made two joints, and I puffed like a dragon.

Suddenly it all hit me I was wobbly and dizzy.

As I went to stand up Annabel stopped me from falling.

She held me under my arm and led me to her downstairs bedroom. I lay down on the bed and even in a drunken and stoned state; I began to pray to the heavens to help me deal with the reoccurrence of can-sir. I drifted off to sleep and four hours later Annabel woke me up.

By now the raging storm had semi subsided.

My head was a lot clearer by now.

I sat in Annabel's kitchen, and I asked her to explain what happened in the consulting room.

Annabel explained the best she could, and she told me that I had to go to the hospital at two o clock the following day.

I had a few cups of coffee and then I drove home.

I lit some candles and I tried to create a holy and relaxing environment.

I found it hard to settle that night but I did.

I decided not to let this incident disturb my mind.

I went to bed early and with my beads in hand, I prayed for a calm mind and a peaceful journey to Heaven.

The next morning I slept in till eleven o clock.

When I woke I felt calm and at peace. I prayed for a short time, and then I got up and washed and dressed myself.

As the morning moved on, my thoughts deepened.

I thought if I had a James Bond attitude, as in die another day all would be well.

That morning before the appointment I had not got the energy or the will to cry. I felt strong within myself.

I was looking at this latest episode as a challenge to inspire me to enjoy one day at a time, and move out of the doldrums of my mind.

Now I understand that I only truly have one day at a time, and whether we like it or not we all only have one day at a time. Because I know and believe this I found it easy and rewarding to apply this principle to my life.

My present state of bewilderment was evaporating from my mind. That morning it felt like I put the predator back in his cage. I was always weighing up my chances, but now I learned to let God do all that stuff for me. My job was simply to live the best I can and to be the happiest I can be, but only one day at a time. The morning swiftly passed by and soon enough I found myself back in Doctors Calvert's waiting room. This time it was full of sick people, bald people, and people with puffed out faces and bodies. The sight scared me but I made my mind stand fast. An hour passed by and I held my composure.

Suddenly my name was called. I entered the doctors consulting room and sat down. As soon as I sat down Doctor Calvert asked me how I was feeling.

With a slight grin on my face I said fine. She explained in detail about my four tumours, and asked me did I understand. I said yes Doctor now can you tell me what my options are.

Option one she said is chemotherapy and option two is radium treatment. I looked at her and in a mille-second my mind was made up, and to her amazement I said no to both treatments. She fumbled around with some paper work in her hands. I was delighted that I said no. I was relieved that I was not going to be poisoned to my grave.

These treatments to me sounded like a death sentence.

Eventually the doctor looked at me again and said, "Mister Power I think it's your lucky day." I asked why.

She told me that there was a new drug on the market for special kinds of can-sir, and my kind fits the bill.

I asked her was it a chemo drug.

She said, "No Mister Power it's an anti can-sir targeted drug, but it's classed as a chemo drug." I asked her for the name of the drug and she simply said "SUTENT."

I asked her to give me a couple of days to make my mind up. She agreed and stood up. I shook her hand and then I left her office. As soon as I got home I popped open the lap top, and I began to do some serious research on this drug. From all the knowledge I attained about this new drug it seemed to tick all the boxes for me.

This drug was derived from a plant source and this naturalism suited me down to the ground.

Two days later I returned to the hospital with a positive frame of mind. I told Doctor Calvert I would be prepared to give it a go. She arranged a heart test, and my bloods were taken. I wondered around the hospital while waiting for the results. Three hours later my phone rang I answered it, and I was asked to go to the chemo ward.

I nervously made my way there.

I rang the bell at the little hatch door, the receptionist asked me my name and buzzed me in. As I entered my eyes instantly scanned the big well lit room.

I was shocked to see lots of people connected to i.v lines and drips, young, old, rich, and poor, it didn't matter. We were all here for the one thing. I looked at the nurses administering their deadly cocktails of poisonous drugs. Some had happy faces and some looked like they were wore out and weary.

Suddenly an angelic faced nurse approached me and said, "Hello Mister Power my name is Aida." I shook her hand and she led me to my chair. Her words were kind, and I felt a reassuring sense of confidence coming from her.

Aida told me that my bloods were fine and my heart was in good condition. My blood pressure was taken and I was weighed. Ten minutes later an intern doctor approached me. He fumbled around with my charts for a couple of minutes, and then he said something that blew my mind off this planet.

He said, "Mister Power I bet you a pound to a penny that you are the healthiest person in here."

He sat down along side of me and explained all about the drug that I would be taking. Before I left I was given an appointment card and a prescription for my high technology tablets.

As soon as I got out of the hospital I drove to the chemist and got my tablets. I drove home, and that day I took my first anti can-sir drug. For the rest of the day I sat and watched the television, and I monitored myself for any reaction to the new drug in my system. I was waiting for aches or pains but they never came. I went to bed at ten thirty and I preyed for peace in my mind. I was pleased that the tablet went down well with me.

When I woke I felt ok. I had scrambled egg and toast and a couple of cups of coffee. At ten o clock I took my tablet and set my phones alarm for ten o clock for every morning for the month's course of tablets.

The week flew by and it was time for a review of my so called chemo. I got up and washed and dressed. I swallowed down a protein drink and my mock chemo as I called it. I made my way to the hospital for my appointment. My bloods were taken and I sat in the chemo ward, waiting for the doctor to give the o.k. for the next course of treatment.

I eventually got the go ahead to start the next bombardment of SUTENT. I left the hospital that day and deep inside me, I somehow knew that the drug was starting to work in me.

After three months of this treatment I had no external reaction to this drug and internally I felt fine.

One morning I received a letter to go for a C.T. scan on my chest area.

It was a very nervous and anxious time for me but I coped very well with the stress involved. The following week I went for my scans, and as soon as it was finished I asked the operator when the results would be ready. He told me in a week's time. My mind was up in a heap because I did not like waiting for results.

Waiting a week for the results I knew would play havoc with my thoughts. When I left the hospital I went and bought a bag of cannabis, and went home and I smoked literally until the night before my scan results were due.

I made my way to the hospital and I plopped myself down in the waiting room. An hour passed by and I was beginning to get bored and anxious and sweaty.

Suddenly I was called into the doctor's office.

I wiped my forehead with my sleeve, and I stood up and went into the office and sat down. Doctor Calvert looked at me and said, "Things are looking good Mister Power."

Instantly I said what's looking good.

She told me that the tumours on my lungs had not grown any bigger in size. As she said this I felt a wave of energy hope and relief welled up inside me. I could hardly contain myself from crying. I left her office and it was like I won the lottery that day. As I left the hospital I had a spring in my step. I prayed and gave thanks to the almighty one until I reached my car. I sat in my car and I realised that faith had intervened in my life again. I felt like a barrier or a blockage had being lifted from my mind and soul.

I spent the next six months going to and from the hospital, scan's bloods heart tests and so on. Most of the time, as soon as I got home from the hospital I made myself a joint or two, and chilled out for the rest of the day.

I believe that at the time this helped me with the stress, and maybe it strengthened my inner thoughts to carry on and find health again.

In my spare time my buddy Seamus and I went and did a few small building jobs, and the spare cash was a bonus in my life, it enhanced it no end.

All my household bills were paid and this wasn't a burden on me. To be honest the work physically was taking its toll on me, but I did not want to give it up.

On evening after hospital I went to my friend Annabel's house. She put the coffee on while I sat in her kitchen and made myself a joint.

As I was sipping my coffee and smoking my joint there was a knock on the kitchen door. The door opened and Annabel's sister and her friend Lilly walked in. The three girls began to chat to each other, and to me their chit chat was like a foreign language. Their laughing was very healing. As I sat there I noticed a tube on Lilly just below her right shoulder bone.

I was curious, for a few moments I thought that it was her bra strap gone wrong and twisted up.

I looked at Lilly and advised her of her tangle.

Lilly looked at me and said, "That's only my Dialysis tube."

I nearly fell of the chair with embarrassment. Over the next hour or so we shared our problems with each other in the most humorous and light hearted way possible.

Suddenly Lilly looked at her watch and said, "Lads I got to ring a taxi for Dialysis." I offered her lift to the unit and she accepted it. We got on like a house on fire.

When we arrived at the unit Lilly asked me to come in with her and chat for a while. I was thrilled at this offer and we walked in together. Lilly and I were met by the sister of the unit, and then Lilly was guided to her life line machine in a single room of the main ward.

A Pilipino nurse entered the room and connected her to the blood purifying machine, as I watched in amazement.

Suddenly I realised this could have and probably should have being me. My sense of gratitude was at a hundred and ten percent. I knew I had major health problems but seeing what went on in that unit grounded me to the floor.

From my prospective everybody in that ward was suffering ten times more than me.

I stayed with Lilly for the four hour session of blood purifying. We had a ball of a time, we were even told to quieten down a few times. Then Lilly said something strange. She looked at me and said, "Tony do you think happiness is overrated." I said I don't really understand what you mean. Lilly said, "Tony look at it this way when we were loud and laughing we were told to quieten down." Suddenly I understood what she meant. The four hours passed by and I could see a physical change in Lilly, it was like she lost a couple of stone from being on the machine for four hours.

As we left the unit my deepest inner thoughts were God if you're listening please give Lilly a transplant.

We got in to the car and on the way home I stopped at Mac Donald's for coffee. We sat in the car park and shared our medical stuff with one and other for at least an hour.

By the way we got on together I sensed, and it was obvious we were both attracted to one and other.

I drove Lilly home, and as she was getting out of the car we exchanged phone numbers.

As I drove home I was very happy to have met an intelligent focused human being. I was tired I went straight to my bedroom and knelt down and said my

Prayers. I crawled into bed and began to bring my mind to a peaceful place.

The following morning I phoned Lilly and asked her did she want to go to Mount Mellary.

She said, "Yes Tony but give me an hour to get ready."

I collected her and we went straight for coffee and doughnuts.

An hour later we were in Mount Mellary.

Lilly went her way, and I went and did my usual walk around the grounds of the Abbey.

We met up on the steps to the wonderful gardens.

As we took a few steps down simultaneously we caught each others hands, and made our way down to the bottom of the gardens. We sat on an old stone wall and enjoyed the late October sun, and the peace that surrounded us.

On the way home I got the courage to ask Lilly would it be possible to be a couple. She reached over and took my hand and said simply, "yes."

When I look back now I understand that the two of us were, and are still very close. Due to the fact that we both understood, that death can not be avoided.

A couple of weeks later Lilly moved in with me.

We had a wonderful Christmas and we even had a few drinks, which was a no no due to the fact that we both had kidney problems.

Suddenly New Years Eve was upon us and Lilly was booked in for dialyses from eight in the evening until midnight.

Before we went to the unit I had a few joints, and my humour was at ninety percent. While in the unit I was told a couple of times to quieten down.

Suddenly it was ten to midnight and Lilly was finished her dialyses. The nurse disconnected her and we both bolted for the door. I phoned Annabel and we wished her a happy new year. She insisted that we call to her mother's house to celebrate the New Year. Ten minutes later we arrived late, and all the fun was nearly finished.

Annabel introduced me to her parents and her older sisters. We all sat and transferred stories until two o clock in the morning. When we left to go home I felt peaceful and calm and ready for the New Year come hell or high water.

Way back in September my son Shane was due an insurance claim he had being knocked down when he was four. He asked me would I go to Australia for a holiday with him. I accepted his offer and I rang Niall in O.Z. He was caught up in his own personal turmoil at the time. He asked me to wait till the end of the month so he could sort out a house for us all.

The month slipped by and suddenly one morning in late January, I received a text message from him saying, "How de do de bro, all is ready get your asses over as soon as possible." I informed Lilly about our trip and she gave us her blessing.

Later that day Shane arrived at the door. I showed him the text message, as soon as he read it his young baby face lit up like a roaring fire on a winter's night. The following morning at half past ten Shane was at the front door with two and a half thousand euro in his hands.

I made him the big Irish breakfast and tried to calm his anxiety but it was impossible. He was over the moon to be going to the other side of the world. As soon as Shane finished his food we drove to the centre of town. I booked two return tickets for a three months trip to Adelaide in South Australia.

We were due to leave in the first week of February.

At the back of my mind I knew I would have to tell Doctor Calvert, and I wondered would I get the all clear to go. A couple of days later I rang Marian, another angel on earth, Doctor Calvert's secretary and told her of my planed trip abroad with my son. I asked her could she speak to the Doctor for me.

She said, "No problem Tony can you give me a couple of days." Three days passed by, and on the evening of the third day Marian rang and asked me to be at the hospital at ten the next morning. I had a sleepless night and I guess that the anxiety of it all got to me.

When I got out of bed I took a shower, and I polished myself up as best that I could. I drove to the hospital, and before I went to my appointment I went into the chapel. I prayed that I would be let go on my journey with my son.

As soon as I finished in the chapel I went straight to the Oncology ward and sat nervously waiting. Ten minutes past and Doctor Calvert called me into her office. I plopped myself down on the nearest chair.

She asked me how I was feeling, and also did I have any side effects from the drugs.

I told her that I seemed a lot stronger since treatment began.

Then straight up she said, "Mister Power I was informed that you are planning to go to Australia for three months." I looked at her and said only if I am allowed.

She said, "I can't see why not but on one condition, and that is that you attend a doctor on a fortnightly basis."

I agreed and we shook hands.

Before I left the doctors office she informed me that I would have to have paper work for customs for the three months supply of drugs. She asked me to call to Marian for the paperwork on Monday morning. I thanked her for her help and I left her office. As soon as I got to the main door I phoned Shane and broke the good news.

He was over the moon as he suddenly realised that this was really happening.

Monday morning arrived in a shot. I went to the hospital to collect my paper work, and I was informed that the oncology social worker wanted to speak to me.

I was directed to her office.

I knocked on her door and an elderly lady answered.

I introduced myself to her, and she showed me into her office. She told me that her name was Francis. I asked her why I was here. She smiled at me and said, "Doctor Calvert has informed me of your trip abroad."

Then out of the blue she said, "I hope you're not offended" as she handed me an envelope and asked me to open it.

I did and I was surprised and a bit shocked to find a cheque for six hundred euro. I instantly asked her where this came from.

She smiled and said, "Tony when I was told you and your son were going to Australia I phoned the can-sir society, and asked them for a one off treat for you." I also explained your medical history and within hours of my phone call they issued you this cheque." I was over the moon as I accepted this kind and generous offer.

I thanked Francis from the bottom of my heart, and as I left her office that day I felt a sense of deep caring and kindness from others. The following day Shane and I did a small bit of clothes shopping, shorts socks and t-shirts.

Later on that evening we began to pack our bags.

For the rest of the week I kept myself busy in my back garden, and I began to read again. Shane spent the week running around like a blue arse fly, and really getting nothing done.

I also prepared the house for Lilly's comfort and security for while we were away.

Suddenly the big day arrived, and Shane was at my door at six thirty in the morning.

The taxi was due for seven thirty. I made Shane and myself some strong coffee, and a cup of tea for Lilly.

The hour slipped by and the taxi beeped outside my front door. Shane put the bags in while I hugged and kissed Lilly and said goodbye to her.

The taxi dropped us off at the train station.

Shane hauled the two bags on to the train, and ten minutes later the train pulled off. Three hours later we arrived in Dublin Airport. We checked in and went through to the departure lounge. Eventually we boarded a small plane and two hours later we were in Frankfurt Germany.

We filled up on Mac Donald's and coffee and waited for our next flight.

Two hours later we boarded a gigantic plane bound for Singapore. I slept for three quarters of the flight but Shane stayed awake.

We had a three hour stop over in Singapore.

When we got off the plane I brought Shane to the sky bar.

As soon as we walked out the doors the humidity in the open air nearly drained what energy was left in us, out of us. We had a few glasses of water and we went straight back inside to the air conditioned airport.

Shane did a bit of duty free shopping, and I just sat on a comfortable chair and said a few prayers, and asked my God to protect us on our journey.

Suddenly we were called for our next flight. We were the last in the queue, and as we were going through the airport security stopped me and ransacked my shoulder bag.

He pulled out a few protein drinks and made a big deal about the drinks. I showed him the letter but he wasn't having any of it. He insisted that he got his supervisor.

Five minutes passed and the departure area was empty, everybody had boarded the plane.

The supervisor approached me and the other officer.

The supervisor picked up my drinks and said "No no sir you not bring with you."

I swiftly picked up the drinks and dumped them in the bin at my side. The supervisor then pointed to the plane and in a hand jester he said move on.

We eventually boarded the plane for Melbourne and settled in for the next long flight.

I took five milligrams of diazepam, and I told Shane I was going to sleep. I advised Shane to nod off, and I told him if he didn't it would be very hard to get over the jet lag.

A couple of hours before landing Shane woke me and said, "Dad dinner is on the way." I asked him did he get any sleep he said, "Dad I was too excited to sleep."

We had our dinner and an hour later we were told to prepare for landing. We buckled up and eventually landed in Melbourne Australia.

When we reached customs, the man asked us what we were doing here. I told him straight up that I had can-sir and this would probably be my last trip with my son.

We had no problem clearing customs. As a matter of fact the custom officer was interested in my story. I told him about ESIAC. Then he shocked me and told me that his wife has can-sir. I told him to tell her to never give up. He smiled at us and wished us well.

We made our way to our connecting flight to Adelaide and boarded. An hour and a half later we landed.

We collected our bags and made our way to the front of the airport.

I looked around for Niall and at the same time he was looking around for us. I could see no sign of him anywhere. I bought a couple of coffees, and Shane and I made our way to the main door of the airport.

I lit a cigarette and as soon as I took my first puff I heard a loud voice behind me saying, "Hello brother Tony."

Chapter Thirty-Two:

Oz

I turned on my heels, and greeted my buddy.

Niall looked at Shane and said, "O my God its being ten years since I have seen you Shane."

He then looked at me and said, "Tony your little boy has grown up." I just replied thank God and his blessed mother.

Niall hauled our bags to his Hi-lux truck and we all got in. When we left the airport Shane quickly fell to sleep. Niall drove straight to the beach. As soon as he stopped the truck he produced two Joints from his shirt pocket and handed me one.

We sat on the soft sand and we puffed our joints.

Niall asked me about my medical stuff. I gave him a brief update of the situation. Then he said, "Tony if any thing goes wrong I will bring you or Shane straight to my doctor, and by the way his practice is only ten minutes from where we will be living." I looked at him and said buddy I appreciate your concern but nothing will go wrong. We finished our smoke and we returned to the truck.

Niall drove for a good twenty minutes and suddenly we stopped for coffee and cakes. Niall passed me five dollars in change from the centre console of the truck and asked me to get the coffee and three apple slices.

I entered the cake shop and basically the place was a sea of pink cakes and buns. I found this strange. My curiosity forced me to ask the girl behind the counter what all the pink cakes were for. The girl said that, "Once a week we and our other chains do pink for can-sir."

As I walked out of the shop I thought what a good race of people. I jumped back in the truck and five minutes later we were driving up a driveway to a big posh looking wooden house. Instantly I said Niall who lives here.

"We do" was his answer. Shane was still fast asleep and snoring for Ireland. Niall took our bags out and brought them into the house. I woke Shane up and told him that we were here. Shane looked at me and said, "Dad I am knackered." We went into the house and Niall showed Shane and me our bedrooms. My bedroom was as big as my whole little house back in Ireland, and Shane's wasn't much smaller. Shane went to bed straight away; I advised him that if he did it would take him ages to brush off the jet lag. He ignored my advice, and for the next three days he drifted in and out of sleep until eventually he shook off his jet lag. In the mean time Niall and I were catching up on things. Suddenly I realised I had a six pack of Tayto crisps and a half dozen blaas in my bag. I took them out and gave them to, Niall his eyes popped in his head. He quickly made his way to the kitchen and without speaking he put the blaas in the microwave.
He stuffed his face until the blaas and Tayto were all gone.
Then he thanked me for the Irish food.

I asked Niall about a bit of weed and was it possible to get some. He just said, "Come with me."
We walked down the steps of the house and went into the garage. His tools were all over the place and his one thousand c.c. motor bike was in the middle of the large mess. He picked up a large twenty litre bucket and flung it at me. I grabbed it and opened it.

The bucket was full of cannabis. I said Niall that's a lot of weed. He looked at me and said, "That's all organic and it's yours, and see can you finish it before you go home."

I was blown away by his generosity.
We sat on the porch for the rest of that evening and puffed down joints like smoking dragons.

By bed time I was twisted and I fell into bed and began to pray, and I asked the Higher Power to give me a break from the thoughts and feelings and emotions of can-sir.

In the morning Niall woke me and said, "The big Irish is sizzling away Tony." I got out of bed and woke Shane up, and I told him to have a shower before breakfast. We finished our food and as predicted Shane went back to bed. The first three days there were probably the best days I had in donkey's years.

I asked Niall when we were going to start some work.

He looked at me and said, "Are you crazy man its forty degrees out their as a matter of fact Tony we are in the middle of a heat wave." He told me that the temperature recently has broken all the previous records.

Over the next two weeks we stayed indoors and put the air conditioning on full blast.

Every night I Skyped Lilly and we chatted for hours on end. After the sweltering heat had dissipated Niall decided to go back to work. He asked me straight up would I be able to handle a day's work. I told him that it wouldn't be a problem. By this time Shane was in good form. One evening Niall and I went to look at a plastering job on the outskirts of Adelaide. We surveyed the work together and Niall said, "Tony are you up for it."

I said no bother brother; I could do that with one hand tied behind my back. He said, "Ok we start at eight in the morning."

When I went to bed that night I prayed and asked for the strength to do my job which I had trained for six years, back in the early eighty's.

The following morning my alarm beeped at seven o

Clock. I got out of bed and went in for a cold shower.

As soon as I was finished I brewed some coffee and sat out side in the early morning sun. I waited for the boys to rise but there were no signs of life. It was getting close to nine o clock so I woke Niall up and told him that we were late for work. In his half awake mood he laughed at me and said, "Were in no hurry Tony just chill out for your self man." I put some more coffee on and I made a joint, I sat out side and slowly smoked it.

At half past nine Niall eventually rolled out of bed, and five minutes later Shane appeared with a sour looking tired face.

A half hour later we were in the truck heading down hill for the centre of the city. We stopped at a Dulux paint shop and Niall went in. Five minutes passed and Niall returned with what looked like a big shopping trolley full of large tubs. Shane and I loaded the truck, and then Niall drove to the Job. We unloaded the tubs and Niall said, "Lads its breakfast time." We went to the nearest café and had our breakfast. We finished and got back in the truck.

Instead of going back to the job Niall drove straight home, and on the way he said, "Boys wasn't that a hard days graft." Later on that evening I told Niall that I was running short of cash. He just laughed at me and said, "No bother bro." He put his hand in his pocket and pulled out his wallet and handed me two hundred dollars, and he handed Shane a hundred dollars. He asked us was it enough for us for the time being? We just nodded. The following day I was up at six, I took my mock chemo, and I lounged around until the boys got out of bed at eight o clock.

At half past eight we left for work. At half past twelve we were finished and back at the house. This went on for the length of our stay. Over the course of the trip we met a lot of Nialls friends and we spent a lot of time in the pub. Nialls friend Waddo, our labourer, took to Shane like a house on fire.

Most days after work Shane and Waddo went their own way, and sometimes Shane stayed over in Waddo's house.

Niall and I always went home after work, and we always sat in the shade sipping coca cola and smoking joints. Two weeks before we left Australia I decided to go on a shopping spree. I had three and a half thousand dollars to spend.

On the second last Saturday of our trip Shane and I went into the shopping area of Adelaide.

I bought lots of expensive presents for Lilly and her few good friends. I really thought this was my last chance to treat a few kind people that had entered my life over the last couple of years.

At the back of my mind I wondered how much time had I left, on this green and blue planet of ours.

I wondered would I have a ring side seat to my own tragedy.

The last couple of weeks flew by and all of a sudden we were packing for home. The night before we left we had a big going home party in Waddo's local pub.

After the pub we went to Waddo's house and continued having a good crack until four o clock in the morning. Waddo's wife drove us home and wished us well on our jurney.

I set my alarm for twelve o clock and collapsed into my bed. I said my prayers and drifted off to sleep.

Suddenly Niall called me and said, "Get up you lazy sod." As I opened my eyes I felt a tremendous pressure in my head, vibrating with the beat of my heart. I got out of bed and had a cold shower, and freshened up for the long journey home.

Shane put the bags in the truck and as he did, Niall asked him to stay and start his apprenticeship with him.

I was delighted for Shane but he refused.

We made our way to the airport and as we were parting, I felt sad for to think that this would be the last time that I would see my true buddy.

We hugged each other and then we went through to the departure lounge.

It was a long tiring and boring trip home Shane slept most of the way. I on the other hand had medical stuff on my mind, and I found it impossible to sleep.

As I travelled I felt a sense of weariness and confusion. I felt I was going home to slowly die.

After a couple of hours of stinking thinking I took my beads out and I began to talk to my maker.

I asked for some enthusiasm to fight for victory over my condition. As I sat on the plane I realised that my mind was in a constant state of learning, learning to deal with the thoughts of death and possibly over come my Can-sir some day.

It was clear to me now that the answers were inside me, and that power within me could direct my health in the right direction. Now it seemed like that I had wasted too much time on negative thoughts.

I know now that negative thoughts lead to a disturbed mind, and in turn it disturbs the spirit.

By now the engulfed feeling of desperation had lifted from my mind, and I felt settled and centred in my self. I felt ready to accept today in order to enjoy tomorrow.

Our last plane landed in Dublin and we cleared customs, and as I walked through I could see Lilly on the other side.

I hugged her to bits and kissed her all over her face until she told me to stop. We made our way to the train station and three hours later we arrived home.

Chapter Thirty-Three: Home Again

Shane went straight to his mother's house, and I didn't hear from him for the next three days. Lilly and I sat and talked for a while. As I sat there I realised that Lilly's whole physical look had changed in three months while we were away. To me she looked like somebody that was near the end.

Basically she looked like a bundle of skin and bone. It took a couple of days to fully come round. As I did I realised that if Lilly didn't get a kidney transplant, she probably would be dead by Christmas.

Two weeks later I received a letter from the hospital for scans of my chest area. The appointment came and went. A week later I received an appointment for Doctor Calvert. This time waiting I controlled my anxiety and fear.

The morning of the appointment I had lots of coffee and cigarettes. I felt nervous but I was in a good frame of mind. I made my way to the hospital and joined the long queue in the back corridor.

I played games on my cell phone to occupy the waiting time.

Suddenly my name was called and I stood up.

The nurse did my blood pressure and weighed me.

She told me that every thing was fine, and then she put me in another queue.

Ten minutes passed and suddenly Doctor Calvert was calling me in to her office. I remained calm and sat down opposite her. The first thing she said was, "Mister Power I have some good news."

My brain stood to attention and I intensely listened to what she had to say.

She told me that the four tumours in my lungs had calcified. I said what does that mean.

She looked at me and said, "It means that they are not active and they kind of turned to stone, and I don't think there a threat to your health any more." Inside I was bubbling with happiness; her statement meant I probably had a couple of years left.

Out of the blue she asked me how many times I went to the doctor while I was away.

When I told her that I didn't see a doctor in three months her whole mood changed. That day she gave me a proper dressing down and in hind sight rightly so. As I left her office she said, "Keep up the good work Mister Power." When I got into my car a wave of relief shrouded me. I felt like I was after winning the lottery but in my case the lottery was my life.

As I drove home I thanked God and his blessed Mother for just being alive.

I spent a lot of the next three months in the country side trying to connect with nature, and also at the beaches of Waterford. I also read a lot of books on angels and healing and herbs that heal. I also began to write poetry early in the mornings.

Lilly was disturbed by my cannabis smoking and my wandering off at will.

Eventually Lilly had enough of my odd behaviour.

One morning I went to do a bit of work with my friend Seamus. Before I left my house I asked Lilly was she ok. In a groggy low voice she said, "Yes"

I sat on the edge of the bed and began to rub her eye brow. She fell asleep again, and I went off to work. That morning I had a strange gut feeling inside me.

At ten o clock I told Seamus I wasn't feeling too well. Seamus looked at me and said, "Tony you're very pale."

I got in my car and I drove straight home.

As soon as I opened the front door I called out Lilly's name. I got no answer so I called out again and still got no answer. I went straight into the bedroom, Lilly was lying in the bed I tried to wake her but she would not respond to me.

She was still breathing but all my efforts to wake her failed. I was freaking out, and I was full sure she was dying in front of my eyes from Kidney failure.

I had no credit in my phone so I could not contact anybody.

I rushed to my car and I drove like a bat out of hell to Annabel's house. I informed her of Lilly's condition.

She said, "Slow down Tony." Then Annabel said, "Tony it probably a Hypo." I didn't understand what that meant. On the journey back to my house Annabel explained in brief about diabetics, and she told me that Lilly probably went into a coma. Now my head was totally wiped out.

Five minutes later we arrived back at my house.

Annabel went straight to my fridge and took out a can of coca cola. We went into the bedroom and Annabel asked me to prop Lilly up in the bed. I put my arms under hers and gently pulled her upright.

Annabel poured the drink down her mouth and after a short a minute or so, Lilly became semi conscious.

In my mind I thanked the heavens that Lilly was slowly coming round. Five minutes later Lilly's best friend Beverly arrived at the front door. She rushed past me and went straight to Lilly, and started shouting her name out loud. Lilly did not reply. Her friend rang the ambulance and while we were waiting the two girls dressed Lilly. Suddenly the ambulance appeared at my door.

The two men came in and straight away one of them gave her an injection. They put her on a stretcher and carried her out into the ambulance.

As they were putting her in the ambulance she said, "Where am I and what's going on." The paramedic explained to her that her sugar levels were off the scale. The two girls got in the ambulance and I drove behind them all the way to the hospital.

I followed them into A&E, and by this time Lilly was sitting up in the bed fully alert.

The whole incident shocked me to the core I truly thought she was a goner.

Later on that day I collected Lilly and brought her home.

We sat in for the rest of the evening and Lilly explained in detail her whole medical history.

She told me that her kidneys were only operating at ten percent.

Then she told me that before she met me she had a heart by pass to relive a blockage, so she could qualify for a Kidney transplant.

She was really down in her self because the chances of this happening were very slim.

A month later Lilly and I were were clashing with one and other, and the atmosphere between us had changed.

We argued over silly stupid things, and eventually one morning she told me that she was getting her own apartment in the centre of Waterford City.

I left her off to do her own thing, and later on that evening her sister in law collected her things and they left my place. The house was quiet and empty, and to tell the truth I missed her big time.

A week passed by and Lilly rang me, and asked me to come to dinner in her new apartment.

I accepted and that evening we had a good time.

As I left Lilly's I thought to myself at least we are still best buddies. We got on better together now that we were apart.

Over the next couple of months we had a ball of a time, but she kept emphasising the fact that I was smoking two much weed. I accepted this and I tried to cut down but it was impossible at that time in my life. I was truly hooked on the dreaded weed.

A couple of months later I was dropping my son home and my phone rang. I answered it; it was Lily's best friend. She said to me, "Tony it's done." I was confused; I asked her what's done.

She told me that Lilly had her transplant in Beaumont hospital in Dublin five hours ago. I told Shane of the transplant.

I drove straight to my house and packed a few things for the trip to Dublin.

It was Friday the thirteenth of November two thousand and eight, an evening that I will cherish and never forget.

I got quickly cleaned up, and I got in my car and headed for Dublin. Three hours later I arrived at

Beaumount Hospital. I parked the car in the Irish Kidney association centre, and made my way over to the hospital. It was half past ten, and security stopped me at the main door.

Just as I was explaining, Lilly's best friend Beverly arrived at the main door; she walked me to Lilly's ward. I entered the unit and went straight to the first nurse in sight. I asked her where Lilly's room was.

On the way to the room the nurse told me that Lilly was still out cold.

I entered the room and looked at her. She didn't look well at all but she was gently snoring.

I sat by her bed and held her hand. My feelings and emotions were all over the place. Tears of joy ran down my face, and I found it very hard to control them.

Eventually I called her name out loud a couple of times. She moved her head to the side and opened her eyes. She smiled at me and said quietly, "I am alive."

Her smile was the best smile I had ever seen in my entire life, and the emotions and feelings of that event will stay with me for the rest of my life.

I sat for at least two hours with Lilly, and then I was asked to leave. On my way out I phoned Beverly and asked her did she know of a cheap bed and breakfast.

She said, "Tony there is a spare bed in the I.K.A. centre."

I thanked her and I walked there. She met me at the main door and showed me to the room.

I tried to go to sleep but no amount of praying and meditation helped. Deep inside me I was so excited for Lilly, that she had survived a tremendous operation.

The following morning I got up and made myself a coffee and sat outside in the November sun shine.

I smoked a couple of cigarettes and slowly sipped my coffee. I finished my drink and suddenly Beverly appeared and said, "Tony are you coming with me."

Instantly I got up and we walked to Lily's ward.

We entered her room and to my amazement she was sitting up in the bed with a big smile on her face.

I held her hand and told her that she was my hero. I asked her how she was feeling.

She said, "Tony I am in bits but I am still alive."

Over the next three days Lilly improved and began eating again. I stayed in the I.K.A. centre for ten days, with a couple of trips in between, back to Waterford for supplies. On the tenth day after her transplant Lilly was released from the hospital.

I made the back seat of the car as comfortable as possible for her trip home to Waterford.

I drove as slow as possible, and four hours later we arrived in Waterford. I drove to Beverley's' house and, Beverley's showed Lilly to her bed room on the bottom floor.

We chatted for a while and then I left for home.

I went straight to bed and said my prayers, and slept for a good twelve hours.

The following day as soon as I woke I drove out to Lilly and put the coffee on. I stayed there for the whole day, and I did whatever I could to help her.

The weeks slowly passed by, and Lilly was back on her feet again thank God.

For the next three months I drove Lilly to the hospital in Dublin every

Friday for bloods, and readjustment of her anti rejection tablets. Eventually they extended her visits to every month.

Suddenly January 09 was on top of me. Shane asked me to build him a granny flat in my back garden.

I told him that it would cost him the bones of five thousand euro. He agreed and I started digging the foundations, armed with only a shovel and a pick.

Shane and I put our heart and soul into the job, and by early may we had produced a lovely two storey apartment at the bottom of my back garden.

Shane moved in shortly after completion. I was happy to have him close to me, but yet not on top of me.

Late May of that year I started to get a lot of mild headaches every day.

I did my best to control them but they kept coming.

At my monthly appointment in the local hospital, I told a black doctor by the name of Doctor Hope about my headaches. He insisted that day on me having a brain scan. One hour later my skull was scanned.

I was told to wait in the waiting room for the results.

With the speed that things were being done, I began to be worried and nervous and anxious.

The longer I waited the more down hill I was mentally going.

An hour and a half later, Doctor Hope entered the waiting room and called me. I stood up and followed him to a small side office. He held the door open and I entered and sat down. He sat opposite me and in one breath he said, "Mister Power I am very sorry you have a tumour on your brain."

Chapter Thirty-Four:
The Ultimate Tumour

At that moment my whole world fell apart, and I wondered where was God. I felt I was coming close to a nervous break down, and nothing could stop it from happening. In my mind I was full sure that this was it. I guessed that I probably had only about six months or less to live. I hadn't the balls to ask the doctor, any way previously a couple of doctors had being wrong in their opinions about how long I had left to live.

I really don't know how I drove home that day but I did. I held my composure until I entered my front door.

As soon as I closed the front door I fell to my knees, and I burst out crying like never before. It lasted for at least half an hour. Eventually I wiped my face and told myself to get on with it, and be a man and accept death if it comes.

I eventually calmed down enough to drive to Doctor Row's medical centre. I approached the girl on reception and asked her could I see Doctor Rowe.

She told me that I could not see him till tomorrow unless I had an appointment.

In a strong and firm voice I replied and said, love I could be dead by tomorrow. I moved my head close to hers and said darling, I have just being told that I have a tumour on my brain, and I would like to see the boss now.

The girl asked me to take a seat. I did and five minutes later Mark appeared and brought me straight into his office.

I told him what had happened. He said, "Don't worry Tony you bet it before and I know you can beat it again."

He asked me about my cannabis use.

I told him that I was smoking all the time. He looked at me and said, "That's no good for you in the long run Tony, but it's probably good for you at this moment." He then said, "Tony do you remember the bridge, well its time to cross it." He prescribed some diazepam and said, "Tony if I you have any problems come back to me, and don't bother going to the waiting room just go to reception and ask for Mark."

I thanked him and I left his office. I went to the chemist and got my diazepam. I drove home and took ten mile grams, and ten minutes later I was floating around the house as if I didn't have a care in the world. Eventually I lay on the bed and said some prayers to the God of my understanding for some healing. Shit I was really in bits, as I tried to drift to sleep with tears pouring from my eyes. I had a terrible night with twisted thinking and tossing and turning all night long.

When the sun rose I got out of bed, and as soon as I did I made a coffee and a massive joint of weed. I went out my back garden and smoked the packed joint. Five minutes later I really didn't give a shit about can-cir on the brain. For the next hour my thoughts were strong and deep, and pointing towards a positive outlook. I thought things like if I could put a coat hanger up my nose, and rip the dam tumour out I would. I felt now that healing was possible but only if I attained balance within my mind.

When I came back in the house, I suddenly realised that there was still a lot of fight in the old dog.

At that time I was slowly working away at a piece of art work that I was going to donate to the hospital, as a way of saying thanks for all their help. It was a big wooden heart that I carved out of a solid piece of wood that my friend Seamus had given me ages ago. The wood had cracked and it looked like a broken heart. That day I made a big wooden stand for the Heart, and I inscribed a poem in it.

FROM TIME TO TIME OUR HEARTS ARE BROKEN,
CRACKED, TWISTED, AND DISTORTED, BUT YET THAT
BEAUTYFULL CREATION BEATS ON THIL THE LAST
BREATH OF ALL THAT WE ARE, WHAT WE CHOSE TO
DOO WITH THIS BEAT IS WHAT DEFINES OUR FAITH AND
(HOPE). The word hope was not supposed to be on it, but how in the
name of God could I leave this out considering that the doctor's name
was Doctor Hope.

My whole attitude towards this brain tumour had changed over night
and the smoke probably helped put me in a happy go lucky frame of mind.

As the morning moved on I thought how in the name of God was I
going to tell my family and friends.

I wondered would it be better to tell nobody.

I rang Lilly and asked her to come over.

Ten minutes later she arrived at my house. I sat her down and made
her a cup of tea. As she was sitting there she said, "Tony you look disturbed
and stoned."

I replied Lilly your right I am disturbed and stoned, as I said this, tears
streamed down from my eyes.

She stood up and held me close to her and said, "What's up Tony."

I looked at her eyes and said Lilly enjoy me while I am still here, because
I don't think there is much time left for me.

Again she said, "What's up Tony."

We sat down and I told her that I had a tumour on my brain. Her eyes
nearly popped out of her head.

She said, "Tony you're a warrior of light, and I know that this will pass,
you bet it before and I know you can do it again." I replied I (hope) so.

Later on that day I received a phone call from Marian the angel sectary
in oncology. She informed me of an appointment in Cork university hospital
for twelve o clock on Friday morning, with a brain surgeon by the name of
Mister O Sullivan. She asked me would that be a problem. I said no and
thanked her and hung up.

Five minutes later she rang me again.

This time she wanted me to come to the hospital straight away. I brought my wooden heart with me. Lilly and I got in the car and drove to the hospital. I asked her to stay in the car. I gave the gift to the arts council, and the girl told me that it would be assed by the board before they displayed it. I thanked her and headed for oncology.

I went straight to Marian and asked her what's up.
She said, "Doctor Calvert wants to see you Tony."
She showed me to the waiting room and I sat down.
The room was full of sick people.
I waited for at least a half hour, and then Doctor Calvert called me into her office. I sat down and tried to compose myself.

She told me that they all had a meeting about my case and they all felt that surgery was the best option for me.
Then she said, "Tony you must take steroids for the swelling in your brain." I thanked her and I left, and went back to Lilly in the car. She drove me home and as soon as I got in the door I made a joint, and puffed like a steam train on full throttle. Strangely enough as I got stoned the fear and anxiety of the thoughts of brain surgery was eased within my mind. I smoked at least five joints that day, and by ten o clock that night I was flat on my back, with my beads squashed tightly in my hand, praying to God Almighty to make my passing on easy on my mind and body. I kept myself stoned till the morning of my appointment in Cork.

That morning Lilly called to my house at nine o clock.
I was washed and shaved and ready to go. I put my best and only suit on the back seat of the car, and before I left I took my steroids.

We arrived in Cork at half past ten. I parked the car in the centre of the city, and as soon as I got out all I wanted was food, and I mean any kind of food.
The few steroids were after massively increasing my appetite. First I had a big Mac meal, then I had two bags of crisps and a can of coke, then I had a ham salad sandwich, and I finished up with four jam donuts and a bottle of Fanta.

We got back in the car and made our way to the hospital. I parked the car in the shopping centre across the road from the hospital. I put my suit on in the car park. We crossed the road and entered the hospital. We made our way to Mister O Sullivan's waiting room. I was truly shocked to see so many people waiting there. We waited for at least an hour and suddenly my name was called out.

Lilly and I stood up and we followed the secretary to the brain surgeons consulting room. We sat in a scarcely furnished room and waited. Suddenly a short man appeared and introduced himself as Mister O Sullivan as he sat opposite us. My initial thought was this guy looks exactly like Danny Devito.

He reached over and shook our hands.

He looked at me and said, "Mister Power I have reviewed your files, and I see you have being through a lot."

Out of the blue he said, "Mister Power I have your surgery scheduled for next Friday, and all as I am going to do is go in and pull it out and patch you up."

His short few words infused me with confidence in him.

Then he asked me had I any questions.

I looked at him and said could I bring my few herbs with me. He asked me what kind of herbs.

I told him I use Honey, Aloe Vera, and brandy as a natural steroid for the lungs. He smiled at me.

Then I told him that I use Hawthorn berries as a heart booster, and pure organic cranberry juice as a kidney tonic. He smiled again and said, "It sounds like your well prepared Mister Power."

Yes I said and the most important of all is Olive oil and apple cider vinegar. He asked, "What's that for."

I told him it was for constipation after surgery.

He laughed out loud and said, "Does it work?

I replied all the time. He gave me permission to bring my herbs with me.

He then got up to shake our hands, and suddenly his cell phone rang. He spoke briefly to the person on the other end and hung up. He looked at me again and said, "Mister Power I am sorry to ask you could you wait for two weeks, because I have an urgent case, and if I don't operate the man will be dead in a couple of weeks time."

I was a bit shocked but I accepted his request and shook his hand, then Lilly and I left his office.

We walked slowly back to the car and I changed back into my track suit. Lilly and I then had a bite to eat in the shopping centre. As I drove home that day my thoughts deepened. Naturally as one would think the worst. I thought this is it; I am going to die in a blaze of glory. It scared me to think that somebody was going to go into my brain and fiddle around with a tumour for a while, and then pull it out and put my skull back together again. I wondered would I be the same person after my brain surgery.

By the time I got to Waterford my brain was truly mashed and muddled. As soon as I got in my door I made a big fat joint and horsed it into me.

Five minutes later I made another one and sucked it down and I felt I was entitled to.

As soon as I was stoned my thoughts shifted to a blank state of mind, and I felt like I truly needed to be like this for the next couple of weeks. Lilly eventually went home and as soon as she did I made another joint.

As soon as I smoked it I crashed out for that night.

I woke at ten the next morning and my head was a bit fuzzy and confused. I had two cups of coffee and when I was finished I took a cold shower.

I got dressed and to tell the truth I didn't know what to do with myself for the next two weeks.

I was at my wits end so I went to Doctor Rowe and told him of the events of the previous day. I asked him for some diazepam, and like lightning he filled out a prescription for me. He said, "Tony hang in their and be strong." He also reminded me of my previous surgeries, and how well I got over them. I thanked him and as I left his office he said, "Tony on your way out make an appointment for three weeks time, I want to see you then." His statement immensely lifted my spirits.

I made the appointment and collected my prescription and drove home.

293

As soon as I got in the door I took five mille grams of diazepam. Ten minutes later I felt dizzy and relaxed but the pending brain surgery was still weighing heavily on my mind.

That day I got a lot of calls from well wishers and friends.

I had run out of cannabis so I took a walk up the road, and called into a friend and asked him for some.

He gave me an ounce on the never never, and he told me that I could pay for it whenever. I thanked him and I walked back home.

I made some coffee and a joint, and as soon as they were finished, I began to control my terrifying thoughts.

I literally kept myself comatosed for a solid week. That weekend I paid the guy for the cannabis and I got another ounce on tick.

That week I tried to control my weed smoking but it was impossible, as the week moved on I constantly puffed joints into me.

The evening before I went to Cork for surgery, my buddy and work mate Seamus and his brother Peter, and a couple of my close friends arrived at my front door. I was leaving to go to Lilly's for the night.

We all went out to the back garden and sat down.

Seamus said, "Lads this is Tony's party let's make it a good one."

Peter went out the side gate and within a couple of minutes returned with a slab of Bud Wiser, and plopped it on the table and said, "Lads lash into it."

Suddenly Seamus handed me a half ounce of weed and said, "It's a present in case I never see you again buddy."

I thanked him and we lashed in to the weed.

By nine o clock that night I lost count of the amount of joints I had smoked. Seamus told me to slow down but I could not, due to my weak and nervous state of mind.

At ten o clock the boys said good bye and they wished me well. I was in no state to drive so I got a taxi to Lily's place. As soon as she saw me she busted out laughing and said, "Look at the state of you, your eyes are twisted in your head Tony." I thanked her for her comment and gave her a big hug.

Suddenly the door bell rang. She answered it, and her friend walked in and sat down. I was in no mood for speaking to anybody but Lilly, so I made a quick exit to the bedroom upstairs. I sat on the bed for five minutes, and suddenly I got a strange smell coming from down stairs. I went back down stairs and Lily's friend was smoking some pollen.

Greedy me asked her did she have any to spare. She said, "Yes how much do you want." I gave her a hundred euro and she gave me a half ounce of pollen. I thanked her and I went back up stairs.

I had a half ounce of weed, and a half ounce of top quality pollen. I sat on lily's bed and all as I could do was stare at the church across the road, and smoke joint after joint. By six in the morning it was all gone. At one stage Lilly said, "Tony are you trying to smoke yourself to death." I didn't even answer her I just kept rolling and smoking.

My beads were squashed tightly around my wrist. I went down on my knees, and for some strange reason as soon as I began to prey my mind went blank.

At seven o clock Lilly got up and made me a big fry up.
At ten to eight she walked me out side to the bus stop.
We lit a couple of cigarettes and she held my hand.
Suddenly my eldest brother rang me and asked me did I need a lift to Cork. I guessed that my dad had told him. I accepted and ten minutes later he collected me.
As the miles rolled by I began to be scared and agitated. I felt like my back was against the wall.
I preyed in my mind, and I asked the boss above to help me calm my mind and relax my body.
Suddenly I felt a wave of energy enveloping my whole bobby, and this gave me an instant feeling that I can do this. I understood now that I had a lot of knowledge and wisdom stored in my head, but the greatest gift of all was HOPE.

We arrived in Cork on a Sunday morning at half past ten. My brother left as quickly as he arrived. I checked in, and a Cork nurse guided me to my bed in the brain ward. I spent most of that day wandering in and out of the hospital, wondering and worrying.

At five o clock I was given my tea, and as soon as I began eating my son appeared at my bed side.

I was shocked because I asked him not to come.

I asked him where he was staying. He told me that he had only arrived on the bus ten minutes ago.

I got off the bed and walked with Shane to the main door. I asked a security guard for the nearest Bed and Breakfast. He pointed across the road and gave us directions. Ten minutes later Shane had a room for the night.

My mind was now somewhat at ease knowing that, Shane would be comfortable and warm for the night. Shane walked with me back to the hospital.

We sat and chatted for at least an hour and then suddenly he was asked to leave. He said goodbye and then he told me he loved me. I was a bit shocked because I could feel his sadness as he left.

As soon as he left a grumpy old nurse approached my bed and put a fasting sign on the end.

I asked her for a sleeping tablet but she refused me.

I tried to do a bit of reading but my head and heart were not fully committed.

At about eleven o clock I was drifting off to sleep, and suddenly the man opposite me began screaming out at the top of his voice. It scared the life out of me.

The nurse on duty entered the ward and went straight to the screaming man. She asked him did he know where he was. He just screamed louder. She asked him his name, and all of a sudden he fell silent. The nurse pulled up the safety bars on the side of the man's bed, and then she left the ward.

I spent the night before brain surgery tossing and turning wondering, and worrying about the big ifs of the next day.

Suddenly a breakfast trolley was pushed into the ward.

I was fasting but my tummy was rumbling with hunger.

I was starving and I had no choice but to stay hungry.

Time passed by slowly and suddenly Mister O Sullivan and a lady doctor were at my bed side.

The lady doctors took my bloods.

Mister O Sullivan asked me how I was doing.

I told him that I was scared and freaked out. He told me that there was nothing to worry about. Then he said, "Leave the worrying up to me Mister Power." That was truly the slowest day and probably the hardest day of my life so far.

As soon as Mister O Sullivan left the ward, Shane appeared at my bed side. I could feel that he was trying to deal with this in his own little way.

Shane stayed very close to me for the rest of the day.

At four o clock I was given a surgical gown and asked to put it on. Before I put it on, I asked when I was going for the big op.

The Cork nurse told me roughly in an hour.

Shane helped me put my gown on, and then I lay down and I tried to push death to the back of my mind.

I tried to rise above my problems but it was impossible, for I knew if any thing went wrong I would probably be in heaven by tea time.

At ten to five my phone beeped. I handed it to Shane and asked him to read it. He passed it back and said "Dad read it yourself."

The message read, "Tony we have passed two swans on the way to the Tracy Chapman concert in Cork, and I know now that your healing has began, "Sharon."

All of a sudden this reminded me that Lilly and Annabel, and a couple of their friends were on their way to Cork for the concert.

Suddenly a small thin man with a wheel chair approached my bed, and asked me to get in his wheel chair. I plopped myself into the chair. I told Shane that I would see him in a couple of hours.

As I left the ward I sensed Shane's anxiety and worry.

I tried to calm him with a big smile, but it did nothing to the look on his face.

I was wheeled along a maze of corridors, and eventually I was wheeled into the pre op room.

I was transferred from my chair onto a slab like bed and asked to wait.

Straight in front of me were two nurses, one in a green uniform, and one in a blue uniform, they were chatting to each other, and there was genteel music playing in the back round. Suddenly one nurse said to the other, "Turn that music up that's the swan music."

This creped me out big time. I called the nurse and showed her my text message. She read the message and blesed herself twice. I felt a sense now that there was something strong in the universe protecting and guiding me.

As soon as I was wheeled into the operating room a nurse held my hand, and told me in a soft comforting voice that every thing would be all right. Suddenly I realised that I had not got my magic rosary beads with me. I began to say the OUR FATHER as I was given an injection and asked to count to ten.

I only got as far as WHOM ART IN HEAVEN, and that was it lights out for me.

At half past seven I woke up and the first face that I saw was my son Shane's. I was over the moon. Shane asked me was I all right? With a bit of fun in my voice I said who are you. Shane looked at me and said, "Dad it's not the time to be joking around." I hugged him as uncontrollable tears flew out of my eyes.

Shane went out for a cigarette and I lay back in the bed.
The heavy nurse came to my bed and gave me two tablets, she asked me to take them. I asked her what they were for. Abruptly she said, "Blood pressure."

I told her that I didn't need them.
She got angry and told me that she was going to report this to Mister O Sullivan. I laughed at her smart remark, as she retreated from my bed.
Within a couple of minutes the staff sister was at my bedside. She asked me what the problem was.
I told her that Mister O Sullivan gave me the ok to do my own thing. She asked me what I meant.

I reached over to my locker and gathered my few potions. She sat on the side of my bed, and she seemed very interested in my herbs.

I told her that the garlic capsules were for my blood pressure, and the hawthorn was for my heart, and the Aloe Vera and wild flower honey was for my lungs.

I also showed her my olive oil and told her it was for constipation.

She looked at me and said, "Well done Mister Power, its nice to see somebody taking their recovery in their own hands." I thanked her and then she left the ward.

Five minutes later my cell phone rang I answered. I was over the moon to hear Lily's voice.

She said, "Tony why haven't they done your surgery."

I said they did, and for a while she didn't believe me, until I put Shane on the phone. He handed the phone back and Lilly said, "Tony I want you to listen to this."

I listened, and as sure as day meets night, I was listening to Tracy Chapman live in cork university hospital, over my cell phone three hours after brain surgery, lying in a hospital bed. The first song of that concert was called 'neurons in my brain.' When the song was finished Lilly hung up. As soon as she did my phone rang again and this time it was Annabel. I listened to the next song and to my amazement the next song was 'Who Will Save My Soul'.

It was impossible to hold back the tears.

Sharon and her friend did the same thing for the next couple of songs. Then they hung up. Lilly rang me again and said, "Tony did you get all that."

I said yes and thanks.

Then she said, "Tony you're not going to believe the name of the concert." Then she told me that the title of the concert was OUR BRIGHT FUTURE.

I nearly fell out of the bed with spiritual excitement.

Deep down in my soul I knew that I was somewhere within a spiritual awakening. Now just three hours after brain surgery, I felt ten times better then when I entered Cork university hospital. I asked Lilly to thank all the girls for their kindness and then we hung up.

Shane stayed with me until about ten o clock. It felt like he was checking me every five minutes. He was politely asked to leave by the big heavy sour faced nurse. I soon fell fast a sleep.

Suddenly I was woken by a consistent buzzing noise.

I looked all around the room and I couldn't see what was buzzing.

Out of nowhere a blue bottle landed on my bed.

I jumped out of bed and grabbed the nearest news paper. I spent the next ten minutes hunting the blue bottle down. With all the commotion going on the heavy nurse entered the ward and said, "What in the name of god is going on in here Mister Power."

I told her about the blue bottle, and it seemed like she was ignoring me. She insisted that I get back into bed immediately.

Before she left I told her that I needed to go to the toilet. She opened a small press that was close to my bed and handed me a bed pan.

No no I said I need to go to a toilet.

I got out of bed and headed to the toilet just out side the ward. The large nurse stood in my way and tried to stop me passing.

I looked at her between the eyes and said love if you don't let me go I will probably s—t my self within a couple of minutes.

She stepped aside and let me proceed on. As I walked on she said, "Mister Power leave the toilet door open." I just nodded at her and went and did my business. When I walked out of the toilet, she was standing to the side of the door way. I asked her was she spying on me. She said, "No Mister Power its just proper procedure after brain surgery." I thanked her and then I went back to bed. I prayed and gave thanks with my rosary beads, and drifted off into a peaceful sleep.

The following morning at eight o clock I was given scrambled egg and toast and a glass of orange juice.

I was so hungry my food was gone before the serving lady left the ward.

At half past eight Mister O Sullivan entered the ward with his interns in tow. My bed was by the window so I was the last person to be seen to.

The first thing he said to me was, "Mister Power did you do your number twos yet." I said yes. Then he said with a slight giggle in his voice, "Your olive oil and apple cider should be on prescription."

Then he totally shocked me he said, "Pack your bags mister Power you're going home today." I was speechless to think it was only about seventeen hours after brain surgery, and this man was sending me home. I thought he is either a genius or a nut case. Thank God he was the former.

He wished me well and told me to come back in two weeks time. I thanked him and then he and his team left the ward.

I instantly packed my bag and dressed myself.

I sat on my bed and waited for Shane to arrive.

At half past nine Shane arrived. He asked me why I was dressed. Straight out I told him that the surgeon had given me the all clear to go home.

His little young face lit up with excitement.

I think he was happier then me that we were going home soon, and together.

I thanked the staff, and Shane and I walked out the main exit. We crossed the road and took a bus to the city centre bus station. I only had a ten euro note, and Shane was skint.

Eventually I gained the courage to tell the bus inspector in the Cork depo of our troubles. I could see the look of shock on his face, when I told him that I had brain surgery yesterday evening. The inspector walked us to our bus and told the driver to bring us to Waterford. We both thanked him and ten minutes later the eleven o clock bus left the station.

At twelve forty five we arrived in Waterford city.

Shane got the bags off the buss, and we walked across the road to Lily's apartment. I knocked on the door and Lily answered; the look on her face when she saw us was something out of this world.

She put the coffee on and we all sat down.

Shane drank his coffee in a hurry, and then he said, "Dad see you later."

I explained to Lily what had happened in the hospital.

She looked at me and said, "Tony that's freaky."

Lily told me that she didn't expect me to be released for at least two weeks. Jokingly I said I didn't expect to be here at all. We chatted for a good hour, and I gave her a big hug and I left for home. As I was leaving she said, "Tony I will call up later if that's ok."

I slowly and steadily made my way towards home.

On my way I called into Doctor Row's medical centre.

I made an appointment to get the stitches out of my head for five days time.

I left the centre and wandered up towards my house.

As I was walking up Keens road, I noticed Seamus's van driving out of the builder's provider's store.

I walked in front of the van and he hit the brakes.

He stared at me for a few seconds and shouted out the window, "What in the name of God is going on Tony."

I got in the van and Seamus and his brother Peter drove me home.

We entered my house, and I briefly explained to him what went on in Cork. He found it hard to believe that I was home in less than twenty four hours after brain surgery. The two boys told me that they would be up later on. Then the lads left and went back to work.

I was, physically, mentally, and spiritually exhausted.

I put my beads in my hand and lay down on the sofa. I began to thank God for his mercy and love for me. I thanked the lord of heaven and earth for the child like faith, which had being infused in me over the last few years.

Without that faith I definitely would not be alive and above ground. I was slowly starting to enjoy every moment of my life. I was starting to feel like I was living in a mystical, and spiritual, and wonderful, and magical world.

I realise then that I have a lot of trust in Gods love and goodness. His mercy was beyond my wildest thoughts.

I felt like I was going through a process to make me whole again. That evening I felt like I was after walking through the valley of bleakness and despair, and I was heading towards the valley of happiness and hope.

That night I refused to see myself as a victim of this disease called Can-sir any more.

I realise now that I could hand or turn my can-sir over to God for each day that was left in my life.

Suddenly the door bell rang I sharply snapped out of my prayer like trance. Lily and Shane arrived. Shane put the coffee on and Lily sat with me for a short while.

They set up a small bed directly in front of the television, and Lily insisted that I lay there and relax.

As soon as I laid down the door bell rang. Shane answered it and my friend Seamus walked into the sitting room. He looked at me and said, "How is Frankenstein doing." I asked Seamus what time was he calling me for work in the morning. He burst out laughing and said, "Tony the funny thing is, if I called you in the morning I know you would be ready to go."

Suddenly Seamus started pointing to the back door.

I got the message and I stood up and made my way to the back garden with Seamus in toe.

He handed me a bag of weed and said, "Tony I don't need the money for at least a month."

We sat in the garden and smoked a couple of joints together. It was getting colder by the minute so we went inside and he made his exit.

As he was leaving I said see you buddy at eight in the morning. He laughed at me and said, "No bother brother be ready."

I went back into the house and lay down, Lily said, "Tony look at the state of you."

Suddenly I felt sick to my stomach. I quickly made my way to the bathroom and vomited my guts up.

When I was finished I felt a wave of relief running through my body. For some strange reason it felt like the past had disappeared, and all as I had left was my future.

Shane went out to his little house and Lily went to bed in my room, and I slept in the sitting room.

The following morning I woke at seven o clock, and I tried to go back to sleep but it was impossible.

I got of the couch and put the coffee on. I lit a cigarette and went out to the back garden, and sipped my coffee. I looked up at the late winter sunrise, and I truly thanked the universe for its wonders and mystical magic.

I spent the next three days relaxing and recovering and pottering around the house. On the fourth day I received two letters which looked very official.

I opened the first one it was from the arts people in Ardkeen hospital. They accepted my art peace and thanked me for it. I was thrilled to bits to think that my work was going to be on display in the hospital for all to see and read. This letter made me feel like I had shifted on to a different level in my life.

The second letter was from the surgeon in Cork.
It was my appointment date for a week's time.

As a week of waiting passed by, I became calm within myself and ready to face Mister O Sullivan again.
Suddenly the morning of the appointment arrived.
I drove to Lily's and collected her, and we started to drive to Cork.

We stopped halfway there and had a breakfast roll and coffee. As I drove on my head started to panic, I wondered what the surgeon would say to me. I had all sorts of silly meaningless thoughts running through my mind. When I reached the hospital car park my mind suddenly went blank it seemed like it froze solid.

Lily and I went into the hospital and went straight to Mister O Sullivan's waiting room. We sat there for three quarters of an hour then we were called in.
We walked in and sat down, and he shook our hands. He smiled and said, "How are you doing Mister Power have you any problems." I said Mister O Sullivan I feel fine. He just said, "Good good."

Then suddenly he said, "How do you feel about radio therapy." I said I don't know anything about it.
Out of the blue I refused the therapy. I could see the look of shock on his face. Then he explained to me that he and Doctor Calvert had discussed me at a meeting, and they felt that the radio therapy would root out any microscopic can-sir that could be hiding in my brain.
I felt like I had no choice but to go for it.
I agreed with him and I thanked him, and Lily and I left his consulting room.

We wandered across the road to the shopping centre and had our dinner. We shopped for a good hour then we left for home. I dropped Lily home then I returned to my house.

As I entered I became very anxious about Radio therapy. I did not know much about it, and I was some how scared by my lack of knowledge.

I did a quick search over the internet and with what came up, I was sorry I did. My search revealed the possible side effects. Skin change appetite and weight, loss Nausea Constipation Diarrhoea Fever Infection and pain. The one thing that was not on that list was hair loss.

A couple of days later I received a letter which told me go to the Whitfield Can-sir Centre on the Cork road, just outside the city limit. The appointment was for ten o clock that Thursday morning.

Suddenly Thursday morning arrived. I washed and fed myself, and then I made the five minute journey to the hospital. I parked the car and walked into the waiting room. I approached the reception desk and handed the girl my appointment card. She checked it and asked me my date of birth. I told her then she directed me to the chairs. When I sat down I was shocked by the sight of very sick and weary people, sitting there waiting to be bombarded with Radiation Therapy. It scared every single cell in my body. Most of the people there were bald, and a couple of people were sitting there with tumours protruding from their skin. It was truly a horrible place to be, and a horrific sight to see. I could smell the can-sir in that waiting room. It was truly disgusting but I had to push on and bear it.

A half hour later my name was called out. I got up and followed the nurse. She led me to a small room at the back of the hospital, and asked me to sit down and wait. I sat there for at least ten minutes and suddenly a well dressed bright faced man walked in, he introduced himself as Mister Haching. We shook hands and we sat down opposite each other.

He told me that he had read my files, and he was so interested that he had to bring them home with him to study. I felt great energy and life coming from this man.

He explained exactly the whole procedure within five minutes. He asked me was I ok with this; I just nodded at him and said yes. Then he stood up and said, "Follow me." I followed him back to the therapy unit.

We entered two massive lead doors and they automatically closed behind us. It was like a bomb shelter with space age equipment everywhere.

Mister Haching introduced me to the nurse that would be looking after me, and then he disappeared into a side room.

The nurse asked me to lie on a machine for a face mask. I lay on the machine and she put a square of plastic like substance over my head. She asked me to hold my breath for as long as I could.

Suddenly the top part of the machine lowered it self and compressed the plastic over my face, and raised it self again. The nurse came over and said, "All done Mister Power." She took the mask up off my face and said, "Thank you for your patience."

I thanked her then I left through the big lead doors.

As I was passing the reception the girl there asked me for my appointment card. I gave it to her she looked at it and said, "See you at ten in the morning Mister Power."

I thanked her and she passed my appointment card back.

I went to my car and drove home. I took things easy for the rest of the day. I pottered around the garden for what was left of the evening.

The following morning I got out of bed, and I tried to prepare for my zapping. I washed and fed myself, and I headed for the Whitfield Can-Sir Centre.

I reached the hospital at ten to ten. I smoked two cigarettes to try and calm my nerves but it just wasn't happening. I walked in to the hospital and handed my card to the receptionist. I sat down and waited for at least half on hour.

Suddenly my name was called out. I followed the nurse though the big lead doors.

The nurse positioned me on a tunnel like machine.

She put the mask over my head and locked the mask to the table on the machine. She told me to stay dead still.

She asked me was I ready? I said fire away. She adjusted some metal plates above my head, and then she disappeared into an observation room.

The machine made lots of loud and banging and clattering noises. I closed my eyes tightly and the machine began blasting my brain with a radio active substance.

It lasted for about thirty seconds. Then the machinery fell quiet.

The nurse returned and released me from the machine.

I felt a bit dizzy but that was all.

For the next nine weeks I tolerated the treatment in relative comfort, and I had no apparent side affects.

Two weeks later and my head started to be itchy. By the third week my hair started to fall out and the skin on my head began to flake. I tried every cream in the book, but none of them really worked. Four weeks after the treatment my head felt like a swollen strawberry.

Eight weeks after treatment and my head was baldy, and scalding, twenty four seven. This treatment was the worst I had to endure since my journey through and beyond can-sir began.

As each day passed by I felt myself gaining a little more strength.

In early October of 09 I was given a M.R.I. of the brain. A week later I was called in to see Doctor Calvert for the results.

As I sat in the waiting room I wondered was this the end of my can-sir, or would it flair up again some time in the near future again.

Eventually Doctor Calvert called me into her office and asked me to lie down on the bed, and remove my tee shirt. She intensively checked me from head to toe.

I put my tee shirt back on, and I sat up on the bed.

She told me that there scans indicated no sign of anything abnormal in my brain.

My face instantly lit up like a thousand Christmas trees.

It just so happened, that it was my birthday that day.

To be honest that day felt like a double lottery win.

Before I left the office we spoke briefly about re starting the anti can-sir drug. We both decided to leave it go till the start of the New Year.

I thanked the Doctor and wished her an early happy Christmas.

I drove straight home and made myself a joint and a coffee. I sat in the garden for the rest of the evening and thanked God for this day. I had a couple more joints, and it was suddenly time to go to bed.

I knelt down by my bed and gave prayers of thanks to the almighty, for getting me trough this mine field of can-sir.

I popped into bed with my beads tightly wrapped around my wrist. I suddenly realised that this was the healthiest and happiest I had being since October 04.

The following morning I phoned Lily and told her of my good news. She was truly delighted for me.

Over the phone she said, "Tony now you have no excuse for smoking cannabis."

I was a small bit annoyed by her statement, but I let it go because she was right.

Over the next couple of weeks I tried very hard to stop smoking cannabis, but it was near impossible so I did my best to cut it down to a couple in the evenings.

On the first Friday of December 09, at about seven thirty I was sitting in watching Coronation Street. There was a ring on my door bell.

I got of the chair and walked to the front door.

As soon as I opened the door I was pushed back into my hall way. I had a Garda badge and a warrant to search my house for drugs, rudely shoved in to my face.

My body went into an uncontrollable tremble and shivers ran down my back.

Six police men entered my house and I was heavily escorted to my sitting room. As soon as I sat down one police officer roughly slapped his hand cuffs on me.

He looked at me and said, "Where are the drugs at."

Suddenly the door bell rang again. I was told to stay sitting down. Shane walked into the sitting room and said what the f--- is going on.

One of the guards told Shane to sit down and shut up.

Shane said, "Don't talk to me as if I am a dog."

Shane asked the sergeant on charge why I was in hand cuffs. The sergeant said, "We feel he is a threat to us."

With this stupid silly statement Shane and I burst out laughing. We were actually told to stop laughing.

This made us laugh louder.

Then the sergeant said, "Mister Power you have five minutes to tell us where the drugs are, and if you don't we'll ransack your house looking for them." I went to stand up and the sergeant told me to sit down.

I looked at him straight between the eyes and said how am I going to show you the drugs, if you won't let me stand up. The sergeant tone seemed to be getting angrier as the minutes passed by. I stood up, and as I did I said please follow me. I walked into my bed room and went over to my medicine box.

I pointed to the box and two seconds later the sergeant opened the box and said bingo.

He pulled out my small bag of weed, and as he did most of the tablets for my pain fell out onto the floor.

He quickly picked them up, and as he did he looked at the labels on them. He turned to me and said, "That's a lot of strong drugs you have there Mister Power." I could sense that he was very confused. I did not answer him I just nodded my head.

Suddenly from the kitchen I could hear the words "Yes yes." A skinny sad looking police man made his way into my bedroom. He said to his sergeant we found at least an ounce of weed. He showed his boss the bag and his boss said lovely. The sergeant asked me was that my bag. I said yes its mine but you're barking up the wrong tree. I told him that it was an ounce of ESIAC he said, "What do you mean." I ignored him.

I picked up my brief case from the side of my locker.

I lay it down on my bed and opened it. I told the sergeant that what's in here is private and confidential.

I asked him to ask his young faced officer to leave the room. He did, and I reached into my case and pulled out a letter and handed it to him.

We went back into the sitting room and the sergeant removed my cuffs. He sat along side of me and began to read the letter to himself.

This is the letter word for word.

Tony Power
17 Gracedieu Heights
Waterford

Dear Sir/Madam

The above person uses Cannabis Sativa for medicinal reasons. He has had Kidney cancer, lung cancer and more recently had cancer surgically removed from his brain. He also suffers with anxiety syndrome. His minimal use of Cannabis Sativa is pivotal in providing

Therapeutic benefits in light of his medical condition.

Yours Sincerely
Dr. J.M.

When he finished the letter his whole attitude changed towards me. He tried to be nice with me but at this stage I was not entertaining him.

Before he left my house he said, "Come down to the barracks tomorrow, and we'll try to get you off with this." Excuse me I said I will come down but I will help you get off with the way you treated me. I could see and feel that he knew he had made a big Bo Bo.

I just nodded and then the motley crew left my house.

As soon as they left Shane and I burst out laughing.

The following morning I got up at eight o clock I had a bath and dressed smartly. I got all of my medical paper work into one big bundle. I swigged back two black coffees and I drove to the Garda station.

I asked for the sergeant that was responsible for the raid last night. I waited ten minutes and then he appeared. He brought me in to a clean well lit room.

I could tell that he was more nervous than me.

The first thing out of his mouth was an apology.

The first thing out of my mouth was sir I don't except your apology.

He tried to sweeten me up by saying that it was a big mistake, and they were dropping the whole thing.

This bothered me to no end.

I looked him in the eyes and said, I didn't come here for anybody to drop the charges. I came here to tell you that if it takes your name to be on a placard outside police head quarters in the Phoenix Park in Dublin so be it, and that's just for the hand cuffs. I got up to leave and he asked me to sit back down and be calm. I told him that I couldn't be any calmer. I sat back down and I decided to zip my lip and listen.

Then he told me that he had lost his mother recently from can-sir. I felt sorry for him but I had my own crosses and battles to carry. I looked at him and said, please don't treat me any different than any other citizen just because I have can-sir.

Then I told him to go ahead and prosecute me.

He nearly fell off his chair with disbelief.

He asked me was I serious. I said one hundred and ten percent. He looked at me and said, "Tony haven't you enough problems to worry about." Yes I said and every day I worry about Death.

He pleaded with me to let it go but I couldn't at that moment in time. Before I left the room I told him that for what was left of my life, I would always be looking over my shoulder to find the snake in the grass. I asked him to tell me who spilled the beans on me. He refused.

The sergeant stood up and leaned against the wall. He said, "Tony don't worry I know I was set up, and it wont be long before I set them up." Bulls shit I said. I told him if I don't find out while here on earth, I will defiantly find out when I get to heaven. I could sense now that he was scared. He sat down again and this time he gave me the name of another officer and told me to follow the papers over the next couple of weeks.

I stud up to leave the room, and as I went to walk out of the room he shook my hand.

He said sorry, "Tony you'll never have me at your door again unless you need me."

I thanked him then I left the Garda Station.

I went straight home and fumbled around the garden for the rest of the day.

Chapter Thirty-Five:
New Beginnings

Christmas '10 came and went it was the coldest year that I had ever witnessed in my life time.

I spent a big portion of my disability allowance on fuel to keep warm and dry. I spent Most of the early part of that year in the countryside with my friend Seamus.

In June '10 I decided I had enough of smoking Cannabis because lately, I had no life. I needed help to stop or ease my bad habit.

One morning I decided to go to Doctor Rows and spill the beans on myself.

When I got to the surgery he was away on holidays.

I asked the girl on the reception could I see another Doctor. She sent me to the waiting room upstairs.

I waited for a good ten minutes and suddenly a tall jet black long haired man in his early thirties called my name out. I followed him to a small office at the end of the corridor up stairs. We both sat down and he punched my records up on his computer. He sat reading my files for about five minutes. Then he looked at me and said, "Mister Power I see you have being to hell and back a few times." Then he said, "What can I do for you."

Straight up I told him that over the last six years while dealing with Can-sir I had formed a bad habit of smoking weed on a regular basis.

He looked at me and said, "Use is one thing but abuse is not good for you Tony."

He asked me would I be up for some counselling. I agreed with him and instantly he picked the phone up, and spoke to a guy by the name of John.

When he hung up he asked me to go to the Millennium centre by the shopping mall in Lisduggan in Waterford for two o clock. I thanked the Doctor and as I did he asked me did I read books. I said yes.

He suggested that I read a book called
(THE SPONTANEOUS HEALING OF BELIEF.)
I thanked him again and then I left his office.
I drove straight to the book centre and bought the book.
I sat in my car and I began to read the first chapter which was titled, A NEW VIEW OF REALITY.
I was instantly drawn in.
I got so carried away by the book I suddenly realised it was half past one.

I drove to the centre and asked for Mister Davenport.

I was directed to his office. I knocked on the door, and this hip looking guy answered. I introduced myself to him, and he welcomed me into his office. He firmly shook my hand and we both sat down opposite one another. He told me that he had received a call from Doctor John Morley.

He asked me to give him a brief history of my past.
I asked him did he have a month to spare.
When I finished telling my story he said, "Tony what do you want to do with the rest of your life."
I honestly didn't know what to say.
Suddenly I looked at him and said I would like to write a book. He said, "What's stopping you." I said probably fear that I am not bright enough.

He smiled at me and said, "Tony just go for it, any way you can." He asked me would I like to enrol in a class for writing. I agreed and he set me up for Monday morning at half past nine with an English teacher.

Over the week end I fired up the lap top, and I began to come up with titles for the book.

Monday morning soon arrived. I felt a bit anxious but excited. I made my way to the centre, and John introduced me to my new teacher who's name was Sharon.

That first day there I was introduced to writing. I was given a few information sheets on the do's and don'ts of writing. I thanked Sharon and I told her that I

Was one hundred percent committed to do this?

As the weeks rolled by I started to look forward to Monday mornings. As my work was corrected every Monday morning my teacher and I could see improvements in my writing.

Things were going quite smoothly.

Suddenly one morning in November two weeks after a CAT scan I was called in to the hospital.
I impatiently waited in Doctor Calvert's waiting room.
Three quarters of an hour passed by and I was called in to her office.

I sat down and I could tell by the look on her face that there was something wrong.
She told me straight up that the Can-sir was back.

I asked her where it was.

She told me that there were two small tumours between my lungs and that my glands were suspicious looking.
She also mentioned something about my lower back, but at this stage my mind was full, and I couldn't properly take in what she said to me.
She asked me would I go back on the anti can-sir drug SUTENT. I told her that I had no problem with it, because it had worked before.

She made a quick phone call, and then she sent me for an eco gram of the heart. On the way back to her office, I opened the results and interpreted them as positive.
I went directly to her door and knocked on it.
When she answered I gave her the results.
She quickly read them, and said, "Mister Power can you collect your tablets later on in the chemist."

I said yes and thanks. I left the hospital and I drove and collected my SUTENT, and I went home. I was upset for a little while but as the day moved on my thoughts deepened, and all that was on my mind was too get back writing the book.

I must admit that this bout of can-sir didn't bother me as much as before. Maybe I learnt to cope with it better than before. Or maybe I was ignoring it and hoping it would disappear.

The following morning I was back writing and I was very happy to be doing so. I felt like the universe was now working with me, rather then against me.

I felt that my writing was opening a door to a new and wonderful way of doing and seeing things.

I kept plodding on, line by line and paragraph by paragraph, and page by page. I can truly say that my writing helped to heal me, and enhanced my life beyond my wildest dreams.

Christmas came and went and in early February of two thousand and eleven I was heading for the oncology ward in the hospital.

I made my way onto the roundabout outside the hospital. My car was suddenly struck violently on the passenger side.

The impact was so violent it lifted the car roughly a foot of the ground, and drove my whole body into the driver's door. My head violently slapped into the driver's side window.

I stayed in the car and I put my head in my hands.

At that moment I got an instant pain of my head.

It seemed like the shock had depleted all my energy. I had no strength to get out of the car.

The foreign lady whose jeep hit and wrote off my car approached me, and started to blame me for the accident. She started to get very irate, and she started to verbally abuse me.

Suddenly a middle aged man approached my car and told the lady to back off.

In a Dublin accent the man told the lady that he saw the accident. He told her that she was in the wrong.

Within a couple of minutes the ambulance arrived.

The paramedic put a neck brace on me. I was removed from my car and put on a stretcher, and put in the ambulance.

As they drove me to A&E my mind was full of apprehension and anxiety. I tried to calm myself down with a few prayers. To be honest I was scared because of the bang to my head was exactly in my surgery site.

I was brought into A&E and straight away they x-rayed my upper body and head.

I was lying on a bed in the hallway for a couple of hours, and all as I wanted was the results of the x-rays.

Eventually a lady intern approached my bed and said, "Mister Power your x-rays are fine but if you feel dizzy or sick later on please come back straight away."

I thanked her and she discharged me.

I went straight to the can-sir unit and told them why I was late.

Instantly Aida insisted on a CAT scan of my brain. The urgency of the scan heightened my apprehension in relation to my previous head tumour.

It took a good hour to complete the scan, and thank God the CAT scan was clear.

I phoned Lily and told her what was after happening. She asked me was I all right? Then she said, "Tony you'll have to inform your insurance company." I asked her to collect me. Ten minutes later she collected me, and drove me home. I phoned the insurance company and informed them of the accident.

I spent the next three days struggling with muscle pain, eventually it eased.

On the fourth day after the accident I walked to the Garda station and asked to see the officer that was at the scene of the accident. Five minutes later a tall black haired lady officer came to the counter, and said, "You're the chap that was involved in the accident out side the hospital." She asked me was I alright.

I told her that I was fine now.

I gave her my licence and insurance certificate, and she put the details in her little black book.

She told me that the woman who had crashed into me was very irate with her at the scene of the accident.

She also told me the jeep was insured by a foreign national. She gave me the lady's insurance details, and advised me to pass on the details to my insurance company. I thanked her and before I left she gave me her cell phone number and said, "If you have any problems ring me Mister Power."

I left the station and slowly walked down the town to my insurance company.

I explained to the girl in detail what had happened.

I had fully comprehensive insurance and full no claims bonus protection. Silly me I was full sure that they would allow me to hire a car, while they were sorting out my claim.

The girl told me that because my car was written off I was not entitled to a hire car. If my car had being repairable, they would have given me a hire car until mine was repaired.

Before I left the insurance office the lady asked me to fill in a form to claim against myself.

I thought to myself this is crazy. In actual fact I had being paying top dollar for my insurance over the years, and now in my time of need the small print was crippling me.

I spent the next month relying on the generosity of my friends for basic necessities i.e. fuel and food shopping, and hospital and doctors visits.

By the end of the month I was wore out, but I was beginning to feel healthy and happy go lucky again.

After a wait of over a month I was issued with a cheque for twelve hundred euro.

I was disgusted because my car was worth at least two thousand euro. My friend Keith knew I was looking for a car so he drove me all over the town on his big flashy motorbike. Eventually we came up with a small Peugeot from a garage on the Cork road, for a thousand euro.

I was thrilled to bits to be driving again, as I pride my self on being independent and self sufficient.

In April of this year I was called into the hospital for a review and test results.

Doctor Calvert greeted me with good news.

She told me that it looks like the tumours have stopped growing. Then she looked at me and said, "You must really have nine lives."

I thanked her because I don't think I would be still here without her professional intervention.

I spend most of my time now reading and writing, and I keep my cannabis smoking to a minimum.

I am happy within my soul, body and mind, and every day that I live is a bonus and a blessing for me.

The fear of dying with can-sir does not bother me any more. I feel it is more important to live with Can-sir then to die of it.

During the process of writing this book I wrote some poems and I am going to finish this story with them. I hope you have enjoyed the read.

Resilience

No matter what's going on with the sickness
We still have to get on with life and function.

Sometimes there is a certain sense of calmness and peace.

I have no choice but to be happy with whom I am.
Life becomes so simple when you are sick.

When I received more bad news I lost sight of living in the here and
now, and struggled to cope.

But being able to function within your sickness, helps to have you well
again.

As long as I keep doing what I do, I can fight can-sir.
It's about getting up and moving on and the frozen feeling is gone.

The Spirit and the Self

Beyond our rights and wrongs
There is a place of peace.

A place of union a place of harmony.

It's a place where nothing makes sense

But yet it is full and fulfilling.

So when I lie with you, I dwell in this place or sense it's a place where
nothing can be withheld.

All must be revealed in this place of ecstasy.

I dwell in eternal spring when I am in this place.

I was never happier as I cry out into the air
Life, light, Joy and peace, as I blossom towards summer.

Deep within the bosom of the one they call the creator.

So may the blessed spring be upon you,
May it blossom from within the hull of your soul?

And may you pass it on.

Living It

Every breath is a blessing
If I want to survive
I must have a healthy mind
It's a peaceful life now
And in the peace, I find healing.
I'm reaching!!!!!
Towards the loving place I create every day
As the herbs I use infuse my body with energy,
My world therefore is infused
With a positive healing outlook.

Conquering Negativity and Promoting Positivity

I'm not stagnant
I'm not stale
I feel I'm moving forward.
In a happy peaceful way.

I carry all good things
With me now because
I am conscious that
Negativity can be stopped at the source.

My future is in this moment
Here and now, my disease
Has forced my future into
The here and now

The fruits of this journey
Are in all the finer details
Of the written word and
Here is the message.

Store no negativity. Stand back,
Watch but don't listen to the wingers
Plant the seeds of love
And happiness, knowing you
Make a difference in other peoples lives

All will be well.

Lightning Source UK Ltd.
Milton Keynes UK
UKOW050243190712

196225UK00001B/64/P